HEGEL'S SPECULATIVE GOOD FRIDAY

AAR

American Academy of Religion
Reflection and Theory in the Study of Religion

Editor
David E. Klemm

Number 04
HEGEL'S SPECULATIVE GOOD FRIDAY
The Death of God in Philosophical Perspective
by
Deland S. Anderson

HEGEL'S SPECULATIVE GOOD FRIDAY

The Death of God in Philosophical Perspective

by
Deland S. Anderson

Scholars Press
Atlanta, Georgia

HEGEL'S SPECULATIVE GOOD FRIDAY
The Death of God in Philosophical Perspective

by
Deland S. Anderson

© 1996
The American Academy of Religion

Library of Congress Cataloging in Publication Data
Anderson, Deland Scott.
    Hegel's speculative Good Friday : the death of God in philosophical
perspective / by Deland Scott Anderson.
      p.   cm. — (AAR reflection and theory in the study of religion ;
no. 04)
    Includes bibliographical references.
    ISBN 0-7885-0123-2 (cloth : alk. paper). —ISBN 0-7885-0124-0
(pbk. : alk. paper)
    1. Hegel, Georg Wilhelm Friedrich, 1771–1831—Contributions in concept of
death of God. 2. Hegel, Georg Wilhelm Friedrich, 1770–1831—Views on crucifixion
of Jesus Christ. 3. Death of God. 4. Jesus Christ—Crucifixion. I. Title. II. Series.
B2949.DD44A53   1995
211—dc20   95-22988
                                              CIP

Printed in the United States of America
on acid-free paper

Dedication

To Christine for her gracious and unfailing support.

Contents

Note on References and Abbreviations:

The following abbreviations are employed regularly.

SW   *Georg Wilhelm Friedrich Hegel; Sämtliche Werke,* ed. Hermann Glockner (Stuttgart: Fr. Frommanns Verlag, 1927)

GW   *Georg Wilhelm Friedrich Hegel; Gesammelte Werke,* ed. Deutsche Forschungsgemeinschaft (Hamburg: Felix Meiner Verlag, 1968-)

PG   *Phänomenologie des Geistes, Sämtliche Werke,* Vol. 2, ed. Hermann Glockner (Stuttgart: Fr. Frommanns Verlag, 1927)

PS   *Hegel's Phenomenology of Spirit,* trans. A.V. Miller (Oxford University Press, 1977)

Logic   *Hegel's Science of Logic,* Vols. I and II, trans., W.H. Johnston and L.G. Struthers (New York: MacMillan, 1929)

Diff.   *The Difference Between Fichte's and Schelling's System of Philosophy,* trans. H.S. Harris and Walter Cerf (Albany: SUNY Press, 1977)

Faith   *Faith and Knowledge,* trans. Walter Cerf and H.S. Harris (Albany: SUNY Press, 1977)

Ros.   Karl Rosenkranz, *Georg Wilhelm Friedrich Hegels Leben* (Darmstadt: Wissenschaftliche Buchgesellschaft, 1977)

Sunlight H.S. Harris, *Hegel's Development; Toward the Sunlight 1770-1801* (Oxford: Clarendon Press, 1972)

Night   H.S. Harris, *Hegel's Development; Night Thoughts (Jena 1801-1806)* (Oxford: Clarendon Press, 1983)

GB   Georg Biedermann, *Georg Wilhelm Friedrich Hegel* (Köln: Pahl-Rugenstein Verlag, 1981)

CPR   *Immanuel Kant's Critique of Pure Reason,* trans. Norman Kemp Smith (New York: St. Martin's Press, 1965)

INTRODUCTION: THE DEATH OF GOD IN THE WRITINGS OF HEGEL

In 1802 Hegel wrote an article on faith and knowledge in which he quoted a Lutheran hymn, saying that God Himself is dead.[1]   Later, in the famous *Phenomenology of Spirit*, he again broaches this theme. In the end he would return to the death of God in every major work he wrote, save the capacious *Logic*. This prompts the following question: Does the death of God as presented in Hegel's works provide a point of departure for understanding what is referred to as his "System"?

A review of recent scholarship on this theme reveals the following dichotomy. There is a considerable literature on the question of God, some of which deals explicitly with the death of God. Also, there is a lesser though substantial body of material on the question of Hegel's system. However, there does not seem to be even a single work which deals with the relation between these two questions. Let me now present a few comments about some of the more remarkable works dealing with Hegel's understanding of God.

The work of the death of God theologian, Thomas J.J. Altizer, deserves our attention here. He correctly follows Hegel's lead with regard to the death of God: philosophy thinks what religion feels. And if the death of God is that feeling which lies at the center of religion in Hegel's account, so too the thinking of the death of God lies at the center of Hegel's philosophy. Hegel conceives of the essence of religion as the certainty of the being of God. God's being though entails death. Thus religion's highest moment is the innermost feeling that God is dead. Thought, however, does not stop short here. For thought, according to Hegel, retraces the path laid down in religion, proceeding from the death of God to Being. For philosophy, then, death is seen as the absolute necessity. Altizer's theology suits this Hegelian truth well, for it rethinks religion from the absolute perspective of the death of God. And if Altizer has concentrated on articulating and communicating the necessary transformation of religion, and has not devoted his efforts to the correlative transformation of philosophy, this is because he is a theologian. And theology, though radically altered, is not precluded by Hegel's weighty thought. All that can be said is that Altizer has not chosen to dwell within the inner precincts of Hegel's philosophy.

A word about the important work of the theologian, Eberhard Jüngel, before passing on to those who have taken up the task of Hegel's philosophy proper. Jüngel has argued that the death of God in Hegel represents a watershed between a previous age dominated by theology and our present, atheistic world. This is, in my opinion, basically on the mark. The death of God in Hegel does compel us to consider the deep relation between theology and atheism, or as Friedrich Schleiermacher put it, the possibility of theology must be reconsidered in modernity. But Jüngel draws the distinction between these two positions from the side of theology, so that Hegel's philosophy is made to appear as atheism pure and simple. Yet philosophy, for Hegel, does not imply that "God" is an empty word. Much rather, philosophy expounds the logic of the death of God. The death of God means: Being negates itself. God is an empty word only if philosophy fails to think Being in its determinateness, as negation and the negation of negation.

Significant scholarship in the philosophy of religion has concentrated on the intelligibility of Hegel's concept of God, including the notion of the death of God. Generally such scholarship leans either toward an anthropological or a theological position on Hegel. Patrick Masterson, for example, has criticized the philosophical merit of Hegel's concept of God on the basis that it is problematic. He ventures a de-mythologized, or anthropological reading of Hegel, stripping away references to God. But, even though the death of God in Hegel is highly problematic, it is not, as Masterson maintains, misleading to philosophy. The radically transformative language of the utterance of the death of God is precisely the point of departure for the discourse which makes up the core of Hegel's philosophy. The utterance of the death of God would thus be a philosophical mistake only if one rejected the transformation of philosophy expressed in Hegel's philosophical discourse. Quentin Lauer has also questioned the philosophical significance of Hegel's concept of God. His approach belongs to philosophical theology. His analysis of Hegel's concept of God relies upon a supposed intention: Hegel intended that Spirit be identified with the (transcendent) God of Christianity. Presupposing this intention, Lauer essays to show that Hegel's otherwise problematic concept of God is given its sense by the confessions of Christianity. This, I would maintain, begs the question. To claim that Hegel intended Spirit to be the God of Christianity is to say he uttered the death of God in such a manner as to announce and express the transition from inner feeling to outward manifestation in thought. To think God, for Hegel, is to know death as the truth of the world and all that is. Thus, in a sense quite apart from what Lauer contends,

Hegel's philosophy is indeed more than mere logic; Spirit is not simply the machinations of formal reasoning. It is much rather that life which leads from death to Being. If the course of this life passes through the confessions of Christianity, it does not remain there, and so Spirit is not identical with the transcendent deity of the Christian religion.

Those attempts to interrogate the sense of Hegel's concept of God, and especially his utterance of the death of God, appear to be somewhat misguided. For, unless one takes Hegel's speculative discourse as central to his philosophy, the sense of what he wrote about God remains obscure in the highest degree. One of the basic points of my investigation into the death of God in Hegel is precisely to show that the question of what does and does not make sense for philosophical thinking is fundamentally changed by the utterance of the death of God. In short, to wonder whether or how the death of God in Hegel makes sense is not the same as asking whether reflection upon the utterance of the death of God better enables one to read Hegel's philosophy. It is the latter question which I will pursue. And, if reading Hegel leads to nonsense, so be it. But this is the sort of nonsense which must be undertaken if one truly aspires to criticize his thought.

It is the thought of Alexandre Kojeve that comes closest to combining the question of system and the death of God in Hegel. In his profound understanding of Hegel's discourse as a *logos* on death lies the kernel of truth. Philosophy, for Hegel, is to learn to die. This much I grant. The sole shortcoming of Kojeve's approach is his over-enthusiasm for rendering philosophy as anthropology. For death is not the unique property of humankind. It is in fact the meaning of Spirit, divine and human.

Let us now turn briefly to the question of system in Hegel's thought. It is generally thought that "system" signifies in Hegel an architectonic by which the traditional subjects of philosophy, e.g., logic, ethics, physics, are to be placed in systematic relation to one another.[2] A closer look, however, reveals that the matter is more complex.

H.S. Harris notes that Hegel aspired to a system well before he had taken up the vocation of philosophy.[3] This system was a reflective consideration of the course of human life generally considered. It evolved from elements more proper to Romanticism than philosophy. Heart, sensibility, fantasy; love and experience were the essentials of this ideal "system of life".[4]

This early conception of system was to develop during Hegel's Jena-period into a more properly philosophical presentation of the relation of spirit and nature.[5] Hegel determined that this integration of nature and spirit must present knowledge in its totality.[6] He entitled this totality "the system of speculative philosophy."[7] Alternatively construed this system was to display the living unity of philosophy and life in the organic structure: logic, metaphysics, philosophy of nature and spirit.[8]

Frustrated by his futile attempts to publish a work containing this system, Hegel abandoned the project. He distinguished between the task of writing a speculative philosophy and the preliminary concern of presenting a phenomenology of spirit. This latter came to occupy his full attention.[9]

The young philosopher, even while driven by Romantic yearning, aspired to more thoroughly rigorous knowledge. Thus the famous *Phenomenology of Spirit*, though a description of the life of consciousness--a fair *Bildungsroman* of spirit--was deemed a system of science.[10]

The *Phenomenology* was to provide the first part of a two-part system entitled The *Science of Knowledge*. The second part of this system, however, was never written.[11] Instead the *Science of Logic* and, more completely, the *Encyclopaedia of the Philosophical Sciences* was published. It was the appearance of his philosophy in outline in the *Encyclopaedia* that gives the impression that Hegel had finally in view a traditional philosophical system. Consideration of the origin and aim of this work, however, indicates that the matter is still somewhat more involved.

In 1816 Hegel was appointed professor at the University of Heidelberg.[12] A condition of his employment was that he immediately publish a textbook as a compendium to his lectures. The result was the *Encyclopaedia*. The work was brought out belatedly, during Hegel's second year of tenure at the university, and still it was not to the author's own liking. In the foreword he remarked expressly that his hand had been forced, and that he had thus come to present the structure of his philosophy prematurely.[13]

As an epitome, or summary, of the subjects of logic, nature, and spirit, the *Encyclopaedia* is necessarily an incomplete presentation of Hegel's system. Moreover, it is perhaps not even a fair likeness. Charles Hegel, the philosopher's son, remarked that his father used not to adhere in his lectures to the subdivisions of a subject he had once made. Hegel did not follow the compendia closely because he was of the opinion that thought and truth must be liberal in the matters of philosophy, if they are to lay hold of the philosophic idea and life.[14] Rosenkranz in his turn notes that Hegel never ceased striving to discover the definitive expression for his philosophy, and that the older and more educated the philosopher became the more difficult and compelling became this task.[15] The *Encyclopaedia*, then, composed as it was in contradiction to the philosophical principles laid down by its author, may well not be representative of Hegel's intended system.[16]

Finally, even if the *Encyclopaedia* could be taken as a fair representation of the relationship between logic, nature and spirit, to take it as the system itself obscures its important relation to the *Phenomenology*, which must be seen as its presupposition. For without the standpoint achieved in the *Phenomenology*, the *Encyclopaedia* cannot be grasped as science.[18]

Alexandre Kojeve's ground-breaking work on Hegel[19] exploits the theme of language in attempting to demarcate the philosopher's system. He argues, on the basis of the preface to the *Phenomenology*, that Hegel's system is the totality itself of the movement of the dialectic.[20] And, because dialectic is expressed in language, as coherent discourse (*Logos*)[21], Hegel's system is fully articulate only in the sum of what he said and wrote.[22]

For my part I will suggest that the system of Hegel's thinking is partially manifest in his corpus, and yet remains entwined within the obscurity of his language. For his philosophical discourse is incomplete, failing finally to become a closed system, and this is buried amidst the ruins of his philosophical edifice: the books he wrote. But with the death of God as our guide we will be able to exhume this discourse, and present its outlines in systematic form.

Allow me now to recaptitulate. There was a flurry of interest in Hegel's writings in the post-war years. The past 40 years has brought about a sustained Hegel renaissance, so that today Hegel is widely considered to be a key figure in modern, and especially post-modern, thought. A significant portion of the scholarship done on Hegel during this period has probed the topic of God, or the divine. Not unexpectedly, however, recent students of Hegel have achieved no more of a consensus on this point than did the right and the left wings of early Hegelianism. At most we can find some rather stable issues, such as the relation of the finite and the infinite; the relation of concept and image; the nature of death. Scattered throughout this material are comments about the death of God and related themes (e.g., atheism, secularization). Some scholars have devoted significant attention to the subject, but mostly in passing on to other pre-conceived schemes. Nowhere is there to be found a comprehensive study of this topic. The present investigation is a start.

Generally, I suggest Hegel's philosophical system can be read from the composite perspective of the last pages of several of his major works, where the death of God figures prominently in the dialectic of speculative and critical discourse.[23] Central to the present investigation is Hegel's *Faith and Knowledge* which concludes with the notion of a speculative Good Friday, an insight into the feeling that God himself has died.[24] The *Phenomenology* ends with a flourish, employing the phrase, "the Golgotha of absolute spirit."[25] *The Philosophy of Right*[26] and *Lectures on the Philosophy of Religion*[27] refer in their final passages to the death of God in the "infinite grief" known to mind and world. Lastly, the P*hilosophy of History* alludes to the death of God at its end, calling the history of the world the only true theodicy, the reconciliation of spirit and world in the insight that God must be justified through the realization of spirit in history, a realization which entails the death of God.[28] Indeed the only major works of Hegel which do not end with some reference to the death of God are the *Science of Logic* and the *Encyclopaedia of Philosophical Sciences*, and it will be suggested that the death of God is missing in these works only because they represent the product of thought, once it has digested the death of God.

Rather than attempt to account for the death of God in all that Hegel wrote, I will focus upon his first utterance of this thought in the article on faith and knowledge from the *Critical Journal of Philosophy*.[29] As the occasion permits I will draw comparisons or contrasts between this early text and Hegel's previous and subsequent writings.

The utterance in question is found in the following paragraph:

> But the pure concept or infinity as the abyss of nothingness in which all being is engulfed, must signify the infinite grief [of the finite] purely as a moment of the supreme Idea, and no more than a moment. Formerly, the infinite grief only existed historically in the formative process of culture. It existed as the feeling [414] that "God Himself is dead," upon which the religion of more recent times rests; the same feeling that Pascal expressed in so to speak sheerly empirical form: "la nature est telle qu'elle *marque* partout un Dieu *perdu* et dans l'homme et hors de l'homme." [Nature is such that it *signifies* everywhere a lost God both within and outside man]. By marking this feeling as a moment of the supreme Idea, the pure concept must give philosophical existence to what used to be either the moral precept that we must sacrifice the empirical being (*Wesen*), or the concept of formal abstraction [e.g., the categorical imperative]. Thereby it must re-establish for philosophy the Idea of absolute freedom and along with it the absolute Passion, the speculative Good Friday in place of the historic Good Friday. Good Friday must be speculatively re-established in the whole truth and harshness of its Godforsakenness. Since the [more] serene, less well grounded, and more individual style of the dogmatic philosophies and of the natural religions must vanish, the highest totality can and must achieve its resurrection solely from this harsh consciousness of loss, encompassing everything, and ascending in all its earnestness and out of its deepest ground to the most serene freedom of its shape.[30]

Allow me to present a brief sketch of the argument I wish to substantiate in the chapters to follow. In the above passage Hegel associates the critical philosophy of Kant with the death of God. The agnosticism of a philosophy based in the "pure concept" of the understanding is at issue here. Kant removed God to the hinterlands of thought, declaiming any genuine knowledge of the divine being. Thus God became a mere hypothesis of theoretical thinking and a postulate of moral reasoning. As Kant had shown in his famous demolition of the so-called ontological proof of the existence of God, though we can indeed think of God, we cannot thereby guarantee his existence.

Hegel saw in this a great failure of thinking. The critical philosophy had blocked the path to knowledge; it lacked the essential subject of philosophy, namely, a necessary being. Thus it led us to feel an infinite grief, a loss of what is highest, the death of God Himself. At the same time, however, the feeling that God had died was the occasion of a revolution in philosophy and culture.

Armed with a vital notion of speculative thinking, Hegel sought to show that the feeling that God is dead could be transformed into the most profound of all thoughts. Yet this would involve a revolution in thinking itself. To bring about this revolution Hegel attempted a thorough criticism of the then dominant system of philosophizing, i.e., the critical philosophy of Kant. In the course of this criticism he introduced a new basis for thinking, a new idea of philosophy. This new idea went under various names in Hegel's writings, but in each case it represented the coincidence of opposites. Those dichotomies which give rise to the paradoxes, contradictions, and antinomies --to the problems of philosophy-- presuppose a prior unity. Identity, not difference, is the proper index to philosophy. Subject/ object, appearance/reality, freedom/necessity, God/world; these are sundry names of the one true idea of philosophy, of the Absolute. The goal of speculative thinking was to discover the Absolute within the panoply of differences.

Yet the unity of opposites could not be articulated in the language of traditional logic, and so Hegel negotiated a linguistic turn in his thinking. According to the tenets of formal reasoning the subject and the predicate in any meaningful proposition were different. Thus it is meaningful to say 'Socrates is a man' because something different from Socrates is predicated of him, namely, being a male human. Conversely, to say 'Socrates is Socrates' or 'A man is a man' is not meaningful, because the subject and the predicate are identical. Yet Hegel maintained that beneath the difference of subject and predicate lay a fundamental identity: the predicate is the substance of the subject. Thus, contrary to formal logic, when we make predicative statements we bespeak the identity of subject and substance. In order for this identity to become the leading idea of philosophy, it would be necessary to develop a new philosophical language.

Hegel's philosophical language is based on the observation that a single word can refer to differing and even opposed things. In this way language outstrips our conscious intentions when we speak: ambiguity, double entendre, slips of the tongue, etc., all of these linguistic phenomena reveal a "speculative spirit" within our words. Our words tell us unequivocally that identity precedes difference. And this is the truth of speculative reason.

I will argue that the utterance of the death of God in 1802 provides the paradigm for Hegel's notion of speculative reason, and ultimately for his system of philosophy. For if traditional logic tells us that freedom is opposed to necessity, that consciousness is opposed to the world, that thinking is opposed to being, then surely we must suffer the grief of failing to know God. Either God is in us, or He is outside of us. There is no third way. In any case we can only think God subjectively, as our inner, hidden power, or objectively, as something forever beyond our reach. Yet, for Hegel, there is a third way. We can think God as dead. God is neither within us, nor without us. Rather we are without God. This is the truth of the critical philosophy. Yet it is only a half-truth. For to utter the death of God *speculatively* is to reformulate the unity of thinking and being renounced by Kant's philosophy. In the face of and precisely because of the demise of the necessary being, we know the truth of the ontological argument: we know that in thinking God, God exists of necessity.

Permit me to explain. Paradoxically, if we know that God is dead, we know that He existed. Death presupposes existence. At the same time, if we know that God (of all beings!) is dead, we know also that existence entails death. For if God cannot escape the clutches of death, surely we cannot expect to. Thus we come to know what speculative reason seeks to express through language, namely, that God and death are absolute necessities. And, as necessary, they are reconciled from the beginning. This is the unity of thinking and being. To feel that God Himself is dead is to know that God exists by necessity. To philosophize is to learn to die. This is the advent of Hegel's system of philosophy.

Though I will restrict my attention principally to Hegel's writings at the beginning of the Jena-period, my conclusions should shed light upon his other works. As will become apparent in the course of this enquiry, the years 1801-1803 define a watershed in Hegel's development as a thinker. It was during this time that he strove to establish the idea of philosophy and to outline the form of a system best suited to this idea. I will maintain that the fulcrum of his efforts is the utterance of the death of God in 1802. Thus the death of God will be seen to emerge as the comprehensive statement around which Hegel's writings revolve. More particularly, the utterance of the death of God will provide the hermeneutical key to his system of thought.

The following is a survey of the course taken in my investigation. This study is divided into two parts. Part I comprises a thematic approach to understanding the role of the death of God in Hegel's writings. Part II is a sustained effort to read the *Critical Journal of Philosophy* with the utterance of the death of God as my hermeneutical guide.

First in Part I is a consideration of language in Hegel. We shall examine what Hegel says about language as such (from the *Logic*), how it becomes thematic in his analysis of consciousness (from the *Phenomenology*), and how the utterance of the death of God in the *Critical Journal of Philosophy* has a pardigmatic role in his life-long concern with language. Chapter Two provides an account of when in his life Hegel set out to publish his utterance of the death of God. Chapter Three is a consideration of the issue of hermeneutics, or reading, as it impinges upon this study. Attention is paid both to Hegel's habits as a reader and to the concept of reading set forth in his works of criticism. As a whole Part I is meant to prepare the reader for the material presented in Part II. For without considerable introduction into the connection between Hegel's use and conception of language, his juncture in life, and his career as a critic, the *Critical Journal of Philosophy* is difficult and rather boring reading indeed. But, when seen in the proper light, the material in this journal borders on the prophetic, for in uttering the death of God Hegel not only divined the spirit of his times, but more importantly he announced the end of modernity and the beginning of a new age.

Part II provides the basis for this statement. Its principal purpose is to present the outlines of Hegel's contributions to the *Critical Journal of Philosophy*. For, though not all of the pieces have received scant attention in secondary literature, only half of them have been translated into English. And, to my knowledge, no one has ventured a comprehensive statement about the whole of what Hegel published here. That is what I have attempted. My observations show that Hegel's journal articles were written and published in a deliberate sequence. This is a similar sequence to that which makes up the course followed in the *Phenomenology*. There is, however, one exception: the utterance of the death of God in the journal is followed by an essay on the philosophy of right, whereas the utterance in the *Phenomenology* is followed by a long silence, and then the compendious Logic. This difference prompts Hegel's reader to ask the critical question: What comes after the death of God?

ENDNOTES

[1]The hymn in question, *O Traurigkeit, O Herzeleid*, was written around 1641 by Johannes Rist. The phrase, *Gott selbst is tot*, was the subject of some theological controversy in the early 18th century. See Eberhard Jüngel, *God as the Mystery of the World*, p. 64. However, there is no evidence that Hegel was aware of this matter. Moreover, the context of the article on faith and knowledge indicates that his treatment of the theme is independent from the Lutheran controversy.

[2]See, for example, Kaufmann:

> "Let us now consider the system. Hegel had decided long ago that it was to have three parts: Logic, philosophy of nature, and the philosophy of spirit .... The question confronting a man who thought that the time had come for philosophy to become systematic, and who wanted to construct a system, was how to order these various fields of inquiry." (Walter Kaufmann, *Hegel: Reinterpretation, Texts, and Commentary* [Garden City: Doubleday, 1965] p. 241f).

I have given these three parts of the system their more traditional designations, but the difference is negligible for the present context.

[3]Sunlight, p. xxxii.

[4]See Harris's discussion of the so-called Frankfurt-system. Ibid. p. 406ff.

[5]Hegel anticipates this change in the following passage from his letter of 1800 to Schelling:

> "In my scientific development, which began with the subordinate needs of men, I must be thrust towards science, and the ideal of my youth must transform itself into the form of reflection, into a System. I ask myself now, while I am still occupied with this, what return to engagement in the lives of men is to be found." (Unless otherwise noted all translations are mine. D.A.).

Johannes Hoffmeister, ed., *Briefe von und an Hegel; Band I: 1785-1812, Philosophische Bibliothek Band 235* (Hamburg: Felix Meiner Verlag, 1969) p. 59f. For the changes themselves see GW, Vols. 6,8.

[6]Wolfgang Bonsiepen, Introduction to *G.W.F. Hegel: Phänomenologie des Geistes*, p. xvii. See also, Martin Heidegger, *Hegel's Phenomenology of Spirit*, trans. and Foreword by Parvis Emad and Kenneth Maly, Studies in Phenomenology and Existential Philosophy, gen. ed., James M. Edie(Bloomington: Indiana University Press, 1988) p. 17.

[7]Bonsiepen, *Phänomenologie*, p. xviii.

[8]GW, Vol. 7.

[9]Bonsiepen, *Phänomenologie*, p. xviii. It must be noted, however, that it was not until August 1806 (well after he had begun composition of the *Phenomenology* under the title *Wissenschaft der Erfahrung des Bewusstseyns*) that Hegel stopped referring to his plans to publish a work on speculative philosophy that was to comprise the second part of the systematic work, *System der Wissenschaft*. See Ibid. pp. xix-xxi.

[10]Ros. p. xxii. Rosenkranz seemed to overlook the full title of the original edition: *System der Wissenschaft; Erster Theil, die Phänomenologie des Geistes*. Had he taken the important subtitle into consideration, he would not have mistakenly identified the *Phenomenology* with the system as such. See, for example, Heidegger, *Hegel's Phenomenology*, p. 9.

[11]Bonsiepen, *Phänomenologie*, p. xxi.

[12]GB p. 119.

[13]Hegel puts it thus:

> "The need to give to my listeners a thematic guide for my philosophical lectures is the principal reason for my allowing this overview of the entire range of philosophy to see the light of day sooner than would have been my intention."

See SW, Vol. 6 p. 3.

[14]*Georg Wilhelm Friedrich Hegel: The Philosophy of History*, preface by Charles Hegel, trans. and preface by J. Sibree, intro. by C.J. Friedrich (New York: Dover Publications, Inc., 1956) p. xiii.

[15]Ros. p. 17.

[16]Furthermore, in 1831 Hegel still seemed to embrace the two-part system of his thought in which the *Encyclopaedia*, in whatever of its forms, would represent only the second part:

> "This title [*System of Knowledge*, i.e. the two-part system] will not be given to the second edition [of the *Phenomenology*], which will come out next Easter.--Instead of the projected Second Part (mentioned in the sentences that follow above [in the preface to the First Edition of the *Logic*]) containing all the rest of the philosophical sciences, I have since brought out the *Encyclopaedia of the Philosophical Sciences*, which last year was in its third edition."

See *Logic*, Vol. 1, p. 37, footnote 1. It could be argued that this comment goes against my suggestion: Hegel could be saying that the *Encyclopaedia* will replace the two-part system with its threefold presentation of the philosophical sciences. However, even in the introduction to the *Encyclopaedia* itself, Hegel imparts that the encyclopedic arrangement of philosophy is only an expedient. The true form of philosophy, he maintains, would express the totality of philosophy rather than its parts. But just such totality is the conclusion of the *Phenomenology*. It is likely then that, since Hegel had not written the second part of the two-part system as it should have been written, he was willing to let the *Encyclopaedia* stand in its place. For his comments about the proper form of philosophy (totality) see, SW, Vol. 6, p. 29f.

[17]Heidegger, *Hegel's Phenomenology of Spirit*, p. 8f.

[18]As much is clear from Hegel's comments from the *Logic*, which became the first part of the *Encyclopaedia*:

> "Consciousness, as manifested Spirit which as it develops frees itself from its immediacy and external concretions, becomes Pure Knowing, which takes as object of its knowing those pure essentialities as they are in and for themselves." (Logic p. 37).

And again:

> "In the *Phenomenology of Spirit* (Bamberg and Würzburg, 1807) I have set forth the movement of consciousness, from the first crude opposition between itself and the Object, up to absolute knowledge. This process goes through all forms of the *relation of thought to its object*, and reaches the *Concept of Science* as its result." (Ibid. p. 59).

[19]Alexandre Kojeve, *Introduction al la lecture de Hegel*.

[20]Kojeve puts it as follows: "'Science' or 'System' signifies in Hegel the adequate, and therefore *circular*, description of the completed or *closed* totality of the real dialectical movement." (Kojeve, "The Idea of Death in the Philosophy of Hegel," p. 118). Kojeve's emphasis upon the "circular" and the "closed" in Hegel's dialectic underscores that the end of the system is its beginning.

[21]Ibid. p. 117:

"The True, or Being-revealed-through-discourse, is a *Totality*, that is, the sum-total of a creative or dialectical *movement*, which produces Discourse in the midst of Being."

[22]Ibid. p. 123:

"Now this 'Science' [Hegel's system] is nothing else but Hegelian philosophy, which appeared in the midst of the natural World at the end of the historical becoming of Man."

The relation between written and spoken words and his system is as follows, according to Kojeve:

"Man does not reveal instantaneously, as in a lightning-flash, the totality of the real: He does not grasp that totality in a single concept-word. He reveals one by one, by isolated words or partial discourses, the elements constitutive of the totality, by *separating* them from it in order to be able to do so; and it is only the sum total of his discourse, extended in time, that can reveal the total, indeed the simultaneous, reality." (Ibid. p. 126).

Hegel's words in particular express the totality of the system: "In philosophizing, Hegel must therefore above all give an account of his own philosophical discourse." (Ibid. p. 125). Kojeve, however, does not state specifically whether Hegel's words themselves are the necessary articulation of the system or a merely contingent form of that articulation. But, as will become clear in subsequent consideration of this matter, the Hegelian philosophy strives to account for the necessity of what appears as contingent. Kojeve's comments are generally in keeping with this basic notion, and so it is correct at least in principle to read him as I have.

[23]The method and research of my enquiry is based upon an application of Donald Phillip Verene's thesis in *Hegel's Recollection.* Verene argues that Hegel's *Phenomenology* can best be understood by reading it from the perspective of its final page, and remembering in sequence the discursus of the text.

[24]The passage in question will be quoted at length in the following pages.

[25]Again, for the sake of initial clarity, the English translation is given:

"The *goal*, Absolute Knowing, or Spirit that knows itself as Spirit, has for its path the recollection of the Spirits as they are in themselves and as they accomplish the organization of their realm. Their preservation, regarded from the side of their free existence appearing in the form of contingency, is History; but regarded from the side of their [philosophically] comprehended organization, it is the Science of Knowing in the sphere of appearance: the two together, comprehended History, form alike the inwardizing and the Calvary of absolute Spirit, the actuality, truth, and certainty of his throne, without which he would be lifeless and alone. Only from the chalice of this realm of spirits foams forth for Him his own infinitude." (PS p. 493).

The material in brackets is that of the translator, A.V. Miller.

[26]Hegel refers to the effect of the death of God upon the modern Germanic realm:

> "Mind and its world are thus both alike lost and plunged in the infinite grief
> of that fate for which a people, the Jewish people, was held in readiness.
> Mind is here pressed back upon itself in the extreme of its absolute negativity.
> This is the absolute turning point; mind rises out of this situation and grasps
> the infinite positivity of this its inward character, i.e. it grasps the principle of
> the unity of the divine nature and the human, the reconciliation of objective
> truth and freedom as the truth and freedom appearing within self-consciousness
> and subjectivity, a reconciliation with the fulfillment of which the principle
> of the north, the principle of the Germanic peoples, has been entrusted."
> (*Hegel's Philosophy of Right*, trans. T.M. Knox [Oxford University Press,
> 1967] p. 222).

The translator adds in a note that the reference to infinite grief has the following significance:

> "*unendlichen Schmerz*: by these words here as elsewhere (e.g. Werke, i. 157)
> [i.e. *Glauben und Wissen*] Hegel refers to the Crucifixion, 'the feeling that
> God is dead.'" (Ibid. p. 375f).

Though I think Knox is wrong to identify the reference to the death of God with the Crucifixion alone, he is correct in noting the connecting theme of the two works in question.
[27]In the closing passages of this work Hegel alludes to the significance of the death of God to modernity:

> "When the Gospel is no longer preached to the poor, when the salt has lost its
> savour, and all the foundations have been tacitly removed, then the people,
> for whose ever solid reason truth can exist only in a pictorial conception, no
> longer know how to assist the impulses and emotions they feel within them.
> They are nearest to the condition of infinite sorrow; ..." (*Lectures on the
> Philosophy of Religion*, 3 vols., trans., E.B. Speirs and J. Burdon Sanderson
> [New York: Humanities Press, 1974] 3:150).

[28]See *The Philosophy of History*, ed. Charles Hegel, trans. J. Sibree (New York: Dover, 1956) p. 457:

> That the History of the World, with all the changing scenes which its annals
> present, is this process of development and the realization of Spirit--this is
> the true *Theodicaea*, the justification of God in History. Only this insight can
> reconcile Spirit with the History of the World--viz., that what has happened,
> and is happening every day, is not only not "without God," but is essentially
> His Work.

[29]*Kritisches Journal der Philosophie*, Vol. 1 and 2, ed. F.W.J. Schelling and G.W.F. Hegel (Tübingen: Cotta, 1802-03). For critical editions of the journal see SW, Vol. 1, pp. 169-537 and GW, Vol. 4, pp. 113-500.
[30]*Faith*, p. 190f. The material provided in brackets is the addition of the translators.

PART ONE: LANGUAGE, LIFE, AND LEARNING

The analysis of Hegel's utterance of the death of God may be distributed under three headings: language, life, and learning. Under the first falls the problem of Hegel's unique style as an author and the underlying conception of language which informs his characteristic prose. Second is the issue of Hegel's development as a thinker, especially as regards the significant change he underwent in choosing to be a philosopher. Finally there is the matter of Hegel's interpretation of culture, and particulary philosophical culture, as that process which seeks to bring learning to life through special forms of language. To anticipate, we will see how Hegel's lifelong interest in the problems and promise of language was shaped definitively when he ventured that thinking must begin with the hard saying, God Himself is dead.

1

LANGUAGE: HEGEL'S UTTERANCE OF THE DEATH OF GOD.

The death of God in Hegel is not a strictly conceptual matter, nor does it have properly to do with an empirical matter. It is much rather an affair of language. The utterance (*Ausserung*) is a word, hovering between thought and thing, bringing to speech a fascinating, topsy-turvy land of speculative truth and reality (*Wahrheit*). Here life thrives on the give and take between the world as we see (that is, both conceive and sense) it and what we can say about it. In this land nothing is real and true, save that which belongs at once to the world about us and to the realm of words. Brute facts and mere ideas, therefore, are unwelcome here. Such can only be half-truths, the whole being found only in that which is at once half fact and half idea, namely, a word. Truth and reality in the proper Hegelian sense is a phenomenon, and a phenomenon brought to speech.

The utterance of the death of God is a paradigm of the land of speculative truth and reality. For, as Kant noted, God is a mere idea, and, as we all know, death is the brutest of facts. To say that God is dead is to express the identity of idea and fact, and to do so in such a way as to emphasize that they are identical only when they are conjoined in an utterance. Admitting this is tantamount to establishing the absolute priority of language in philosophy. It is to revolutionize thinking by turning it inward upon its own speech.

Hegel set this "immanent critique" as his task because he had come to know that there is no thinking nor life before they are spoken. For the philosopher knows even the wise Socrates' life was not worth living until it had been examined in the unique and moving words of his apology before the Athenian Senate.

The Problem of Logic

In 1812 Hegel decried the state of metaphysics in the philosophy of his native Germany. Kant had won the day, and his doctrine that understanding cannot

3

go beyond experience intoned a death knell for speculative thinking. The period's intense occupation with the pragmatic affair of pedagogy supported this modest wisdom. Metaphysics was generally made out to be the idle fancy of those inclined to shirk their civic duty. Philosophy thus played into the hand of common sense, demanding that great and small minds alike put aside their vain pursuits of Truth.

Hegel carried the banner of the Kantian cause for a time, defending the true, practical vocation of reason.[1] Enlightenment, Morality, and Edification were Hegel's bywords early on. When the magnificent failure of the French Revolution stared him in the face, however, he dissented. He became more theoretical, shifting the balance of his interest from ethics and politics to philosophy:

> If it is a remarkable thing when a nation finds that its Constitutional Theory, its customary ways of thinking and feeling, its ethical habits and traditional virtues, have become inapplicable, it is certainly not less remarkable when a nation loses its Metaphysic, when the intellect occupying itself with its own pure essence, has no longer any real existence in the thought of the nation.[2]

It cannot be said against Hegel that these are the words of an itinerant speculator. At the time this was written he was midway through an eight year stint as principal of the Gymnasium at Nürnberg. Responsible both for teaching philosophy in the classroom and for the school's curriculum,[3] he had recently wed, and generally was on course to fulfilling his civic duty.

And yet Hegel had some years previously[4] turned away from the trends of the day. He insisted that due attention must be paid the metaphysic, which lay in a state of disuse and general ruin. He was not of a mind to refurbish the philosophical edifice with piecemeal repairs or even with an elaborate face-lift. Instead he maintained that the house of philosophy must be rebuilt from the ground up. The changes were to culminate in a wholly original logic.[5]

This was a large bill to fill indeed, and not merely because it involved the monumental task of retracing the course philosophy had taken since Aristotle -- only to discover that no changes had been made in logic in over two millenia, except emendations of the Stagirite's original contribution [6]-- but more importantly because it involved the task of seriously broaching the subject of language and its relation to thought.

Philosophy had failed, in Hegel's estimation, to develop Aristotle's original contribution to thinking, namely, the contemplation of the universal forms of thought, despite that we have in such contemplation "the beginning of knowledge."[7] The failure of philosophy to accept the legacy of classical Greek philosophy for what it was has led to the emergence of a long tradition in which logic has become an affair of abstracting from the content of thinking.[8] The difficult and important task Hegel took upon himself was that of bringing to light after so many dark years the essential connection between logic and metaphysics, learning and life. He proposed that with a fresh start and a modified method "... these dead bones of Logic may be revivified by Mind, and endowed with content and coherence ..."[9]

The method Hegel developed has come down to us as his unique dialectic, a method in which

> *Things* and the *Thinking* of them are in harmony in and for themselves,--indeed language itself expresses an affinity between them,--... thought in its immanent determinations, and the true nature of things, are one and the same content.[10]

The tie which binds metaphysics to life is a newly conceived logic.

> The System of Logic is the realm of shades, a world of simple essentialities freed from all concretion of sense. To study this Science, to dwell and labour in this shadow-realm, is a perfect training and discipline of consciousness [11] ... But above all, Thought thus wins self-reliance and independence.[12]

The connection between these considerations of logic, metaphysics, and life to the issue of language is apparent from a further analysis of Hegel's conception of metaphysics.

The original insight of Hegel's *Logic* can be discerned in his construal of the role of language in thought:

> It is in human Language that the Forms of Thought are manifested and laid down in the first instance.... Language has penetrated into whatever becomes for man *something inner*--becomes, that is, an idea, something which he makes his very own; --and what man transforms to Language contains--concealed, or mixed up with other things, or worked out to clearness--a Category: so natural to man is Logic--indeed, Logic is just man's peculiar nature. [13]

The development of a strictly formal logic was, according to Hegel's account, an error in the history of philosophy which became so pervasive in Kant's critical thought that the formal understanding was divorced from the true and proper matter of philosophy, namely, reason. The result was that thinking was denied its genuine content and therewith its means of expressing itself.

Philosophy generally still has in its thinking to deal with concrete objects--God, Nature, Mind; but [ordinary] Logic is concerned with such thought wholly and solely on account of the thought itself, in complete abstraction from its objects.[14]

Hegel composed his *Logic* at a time when language, as represented in logic, and the totality of human being, as contained in metaphysics, had been sundered. Logic became merely formal, and metaphysics fell into disrepute. The consequence of this event dawned slowly, as a dark day in the history of philosophy. Hegel was thus at great pains to alert his contemporaries to the ominous signs about them.[15]He was ever vigilant regarding misapprehensions of the relation between thought and language, logic and life.

Logic, Hegel notes, enters into life through language. And, in his opinion, certain languages have a decided advantage over others for expressing this relationship. The German language, he maintains, displays a clear priority over other modern languages in the expression of philosophical propositions generally and reason in particular. Allow me to quote this claim at length:

...the German language has here many advantages over other modern languages; indeed, many of its words have the further peculiarity that they have not only various, but even opposed meanings, so that we must recognize here a speculative spirit in the language; it is a joy to thought to stumble upon such words, and to meet with the union of opposites (a result of Speculative Thought which to Human Understanding seems senseless) in the naive shape of one word with opposite meanings registered in a dictionary.[16]

By bringing the different meanings of words together in their polarity, the German language bespeaks reason, the form of thought which is also at once the matter of thinking. Knowing and being are coincident in reason, and reason develops through the multifariouness and ambiguity of language. The "determinate negation" which is language expresses the unity of thinking and being in their very difference.

Language in General

The description of language taken from the *Logic* is true to Hegel's thought from beginning to end. The basic distinction between logic and language helps to delimit his conception of language and even its role in thinking. However, this alone gives a rather limited view of the problem, role, and promise of language in Hegel's career. For it was not only logic that interested Hegel, but also the connections between grammar, rhetoric, philology, literary criticism and thinking.

Hegel was preoccupied with the question of language throughout his life, more so than any of his teachers and philosophical predecessors. From the accounts of his earliest training we know that he dwelt upon contradiction in his essays.[17] This penchant was rooted in an aversion to the tidy rationalism of the Enlightenment and a certain impatience with classical studies. His teachers saw in it only a tendency to employ seldom used and inelegant constructions when composing in Latin[18] and a general dislike for Latin stylists.[19]

The interest in contradiction and unusual diction was cemented in his decided preference for Goethe's *Iphigenia* over Sophocle's *Antigone*. For the choice was occasioned by the fact that Goethe's portrayal of the tragedy hinged upon a certain ambiguous word: Apollo commands Orestes to go to the sanctuary in Tauris and bring back "the sister"; Orestes assumes that the image of Artemis, Apollo's sister, is meant, but indeed it was to his own sister, Iphigenia, that the God referred. Hegel's fondness for this passage was no passing fancy, for in his lectures on aesthetics, delivered late in his career, he says the following:

> Goethe, with infinite beauty, interprets the ambiguous divine pronouncement ... in a humane and conciliatory manner: the pure and holy Iphigenia is the sister, the divine image, and the protector of the house.[20]

His concern with such phrases as express the basic truths of human life was manifest early on in his general enthusiasm for philology and literary criticism.[21]

But, if the written word was full of promise for Hegel, his spoken words presented him with a considerable problem. Throughout his life he would struggle to express himself. In extemporizing, he apparently failed to distinguish between the whirl within his head and what he said, for neither his gestures nor his voice suited his words. Even when he committed his thoughts to paper in advance, he failed to follow his own guide, and so always produced the content in a new form.[22] His awkwardness in speaking became a real barrier to him in the literary circles he wished to inhabit.[23] And it seems this inability to express himself also came to infect his writing.

It cannot be argued that Hegel's characteristic inability to express himself is simply the manifestation of his ambiguous, contradictory, dialectical thinking. The evidence just does not exist for such an argument. We really do not know much at all about the nature of his *speech*. However, we do have much of what he *wrote*, and the difficulty in reading some of this material is directly linked to his dialectical method. That is to say, sometimes Hegel pressed language quite hard, employing it to shape ambiguous and contradictory phrases. This in turn requires that his reader be forceful as well. By forcing language one renders it thematic, and, once thematic, language takes on a life of its own. The philosophical import of this is that his language must be read not only as his attempt to communicate his thoughts to the reader, but also and more importantly that his words must be interpreted as the self-expression of philosophy itself. For is it not probable that his early impatience with words developed into a philosophical genius for language, that what he would one day call the "speculative spirit" in language was once but his awkwardness of expression?

Despite this certain handicap in expressing himself, or perhaps because of it, Hegel devoted more and more of his attention to the issue of language. By the time he had taken up his career as an academic philosopher in Jena, language had become for him a legitimate philosophical issue. In an oft-quoted letter of 1805 to Johann Heinrich Voss, Hegel announced his concern with language:

> Luther has made the Bible speak German; you, Homer--the greatest present that can be given to a people; for a people is barbarous and does not consider the excellent things it knows as its own property until it gets to know them in its own language;--if you would forget the two examples, I should like to say of my aspirations that I shall try to teach philosophy to speak German.[24]

In a less well-known passage from about the same time [25], Hegel had laid out the fuller implications of such a task:

> Every single (person) is a blind link in the chain of absolute necessity on which the world develops. Every single (person) can extend his dominion over a greater length of this chain only if he recognizes the direction in which the great necessity will go and learns from this cognition to utter the magic word which conjures up its shape. This cognition, which can both embrace in itself the whole energy of the suffering and the antithesis which has ruled in the world and all the forms of its development (*Ausbildung*) for a couple of thousand years and can raise itself above it all, this cognition only philosophy can give.[26]

The desire to teach philosophy to speak German is tied to the hope that language can through its magic, as it were, resolve the infinite grief which Western culture has come to know as the death of God.

If language has the power to lift the grief from about our shoulders, it is because language embodies that grief and yet transcends it. Language, for Hegel, is the spirit of culture, and culture rests upon the rift between thinking and being. The most extreme form of this rift, however, is that represented by the death of

God, which, as the negation of the ontological proof for the existence of God, denies that being has its reality in thinking. That language can ease the pain of this thought is attested by its speculative spirit, in which being and thinking are identical. But this is to anticipate that "journey of despair" Hegel entitled the *Phänomenologie des Geistes.*

Language in the Phenomenology

The role of language in Hegel's *Phenomenology* can be distinctly discerned at every level of his analysis of consciousness and culture.[27]In fact language and consciousness are in an important respect presented as coterminous in the *Phenomenology.* They develop or regress in the same measure, and this because the phenomenon of mind and spirit must be brought to speech. Let us rehearse the progression of mind and spirit in Hegel's account and mark the changes language undergoes en route.

Hegel analyzes the first and most rudimentary form of consciousness under the name of "sense certainty."[28] Here he accomplishes two important tasks. First, he throws doubt on the certainty of empirical knowledge, a necessary step in his advance toward speculative knowing. Second, he ventures that consciousness is determined by language, even at its most basic, or empirical level. Let us note at the outset that these two items are directly related. For, by arguing that consciousness is mediated by language, Hegel demonstrates that, contrary to empiricism, there is no immediate grasp of objects. To anticipate, the language which we would employ to articulate our empirical stream of consciousness ends up outstripping our intentions, undermining our certainty, and loosening what we thought was a firm grasp of objects.[29] An investigation of the language of empiricism discovers that consciousness has already embarked upon an odyssey which it had no intention of taking.

Hegel's deft move in subverting the meaning of common sense empiricism works because he has made use of a peculiar quality of language. This is emphasized in a parenthetical remark which comes at the conclusion of the section on sense-certainty:

--[language] has the divine nature of directly reversing the meaning of
what is said, of making it into something else, and thus not letting what
is meant *get into words* at all--[30]

Hegel does not make private mental states, or sensations, or external objects the focus of his analysis, but the words by which such consciousness expresses itself. This avoids the pitfall of subjectivism. Our attention is directed to language as the outward and objective form of consciousness, not to the inward and subjective. This has the added advantage of speaking at once to empiricist philosophers and to our ordinary experience, for in both cases the same words are used to talk about the immediate grasp of objects. [31]One way or another we must talk about *this* object or *this* event or *this* self, and we must do it in a common language. Hegel's argument indicates the implications of this.

The empiricist account of consciousness supposes an immediate grasp of the object. That is, when I am said to be conscious of something, to know it, what is meant is that I sense it as it is here and now, right before my very eyes. The major claim of any epistemology based on this sort of immediate experience is that all genuine knowledge is derived in one way or another from particular objects which are unaffected by my awareness of them. And it is this objectivity of empirical knowledge which is its most attractive quality. But Hegel's argument undercuts this claim to immediate experience by showing that any given object of empirical consciousness is not known in its particularity. Rather, consciousness is only aware of it as some general object of experience. What we took to be certain in its concreteness is found to be formless and vague. Indeed, he maintains that we are not conscious of an object, but rather being in general. His claim is based on a rather detailed examination of the word, this (*dies-*).

In testing the claims of sense-certainty, Hegel examines the use of language characteristic of empirical consciouness. He notes that empiricism is founded upon the demonstrative use of language. Demonstratives are employed to refer to the particulars which make up the immediate content of consciousness. I might refer, for example, to 'this' tree outside my window. I am conscious of this tree as my object. However, Hegel does not take demonstratives to function in such a straightforward way. They do not specify a particular thing, but denote instead that which is universal in consciousness. The tree is not indicated by the word, this. Rather the expression is a demonstration of a fact of something in general --that something, never mind what, is there.

Hegel's point is rather abstruse. It is not that the tree in this example is not a particular object. Indeed it is. However, the 'this' does not convey particularity. The phrase, this tree, includes a general concept, i.e., tree, and a verbal gesture at being. And because sense-certainty cannot appeal at this basic level to general concepts, consciousness is left with the empty gesture. Hegel puts it epigrammatically: "this" only says "it is." [32]He ellaborates his point by showing how the crucial demonstrative adjective, this, is reducible to the adverb of place, here, and the adverb of time, now. Thus empiricism's verbal gesture at being means "this now, here." But as we will learn, such an utterance could as easily refer to consciousness as to its supposed object.

According to Hegel, the "this" which is used when I refer to the tree has a double meaning. On one had it refers to the object, and on the other it refers to me. This second reference is not easily grasped. Hegel seemed to be aware of this, and so he began by scrutinizing the unproblematic objective reference of the term. He asks, What is the This? and answers that it is a 'Now' (*das Itzt*) and a 'Here' (*das Hier*). Then he asks, What is Now?, What is Here? and replies in effect that both the 'Now' and the 'Here' are terms relative to other 'Nows' and 'Heres'. There is, in other words, nothing intrinsic to the 'Now' or the 'Here' because the 'Now' is really only a 'Before' or 'After', while the 'Here' is nothing but a 'Fore' and 'Aft', 'Above' and 'Below'. The consequence of this is that 'this tree' ends up being a 'here and now' which is simply just not any other 'here or now' and so is actually not a 'This', but a 'not that'. Or, to put it another way, I find that my 'This' is not a this in the empirical sense at all, for it is not particular. As such it is a 'not-This'. Or, to get to what Hegel truly says, when we say "this" we do not speak of something particular, no matter how much we mean to. Much rather it is a universal that we utter. When we say "this" it matters not at all that we point or pound our fist or fume, for the particular, in Hegel's account, is strictly *unutterable*.[33]

Once Hegel has established to his satisfaction that the objective referent of 'This' is not particular, but universal, in kind, he proceeds to consider the subjective side of the term. And it is indeed much easier to grasp this point now that we have seen how relative is the sense of the term. We can ascertain readily that the term, this, can have no real meaning unless its sphere of reference in some way includes a subject, or a consciousness. For to say "this tree" means nothing in particular so long as the speaker is not already placed in reference to the tree. The concreteness and particularity of the reference is lost unless the subject's presence is implicit in the context. Now, Hegel says, the table has been turned. For when we began, the object of empirical consciousness was said to be independent of consciousness. But, if the object named by "this" is being in general and not some particular something, then certainly our knowledge of that object is mediated by our subjective presence. The vagueness of the reference when the subject is removed demonstrates as much. The 'This', then, is subjectively determined by the 'Now' and the 'Here' of the 'I'. But, as with the objective referent, the subjective 'Now' and the 'Here' are relative, and so they too denote a universal 'This'. The universal 'I' is what abides along with the universal 'it'. Together they form the essence or being of empirical consciousness. Thus Hegel avers that the object of sense-certainty is co-extensive with consciousness.[34]

To summarize, demonstratives have universal application because they are not confined to any given object, but instead refer to the object and subject of consciousness in general. The truth of empiricism, then, lies in its language, which expresses the particulars of consciousness as universals. But this language at the same time refutes the basic claim of empiricism, namely, that the subject has an immediate grasp of an object, and so it drives consciousness onward to a new level of awareness.[35]

The odyssey of consciousness follows a tortuous route in the section on perception. Partly this is because, as the analysis of consciousness develops, so Hegel's unique terminology and constructions become more prevalent and more difficult to understand. But the difficulty of the section is also partly a measure of the subject itself. Hegel is at pains to get his reader to take a fresh look at perception and its underlying assumptions. However, because we all consider ourselves expert in such ordinary things as perception, he has to work doubly hard to demonstrate that matters are not quite as we think. He plays the part of the sceptic, reminding us that we have already learned to mistrust our eyes and ears. Now he would have us abandon what we know about things in general. Hegel's designs are perhaps nowhere more obvious than in the name of the section in question, Perception: Or the Thing and Deception.

Hegel's aim in this section is, in brief, to prove that things deceive us, and this neither because we are fools nor because things are chimerical. Rather perception as such is deceptive, being not the true apprehension of things, but the far more dubious affair of trying to sort out what is true in the things about us. It is for this reason that he plays upon the meaning of the German term for perception: *Wahrnehmung* conotes taking something as true (whether or no it is).

In perception, it is already known that we cannot grasp an object as a brute fact. Consciousness therefore perceives its object as a thing, a complex, singular object. The thing, in Hegel's language, is taken as a 'One'; not as something other, but as its own thing. Perception, in other words, takes its object to be a unity of given properties, distinct from other possible communities of properties. The language which is distinctive of this act of consciousness, according to Hegel, is found in the word, also (*auch*). For he maintains that the sense of a given thing as a oneness of various properties is conveyed by saying that the thing is this, this, and *also* that. His example is a grain of salt: salt is white, and also cubical, and also tart, etc. [36] The full combination of the properties of the salt defines it, and so distinguishes it in its singularity. Sugar, by contrast, would be white, and also cubical, but not also tart.

However, there is, in Hegel's judgment, a certain danger in leaving matters like this. For, there is nothing singular about any of the given properties in the way that things have been stated. The white, the cube, the tart are universals, and there is really nothing to say that they are not merely subjective universals supplied by consciousness rather than inherent to the object itself. Accordingly, we must be careful to add another term to the language of perception: the salt is white *insofar* as it is not cubical, cubical *insofar* as it is not white and tart, etc.[37]Hegel's point may be somewhat obscure, but it is important, for unless there be some grounds for maintaining a difference between the given properties other than that supplied by consciousness, the thing in question would be a bare One, a 'This', rather than a singular community of properties, an 'Also'. The phrase, insofar (*insofern*), bespeaks the objective difference subsisting between properties of the thing: white is not cube, is not tart, etc. Finally, if we combine these distinctive terms of perception, we can express what Hegel took to be its truth: salt is white *insofar* as it is not *also* cubical, cubical *insofar* as it is not *also* white and tart, tart ...etc.[38] Inelegant as this is, such a construction articulates the play of affirmation and negation characteristic of the dialectic of perception. For, even as we take something to be true, we know that it is not the truth; the very tentativeness of our speech conveys our reservation. The salt is white, is cubical, is tart. Yet, at the same time, it is neither the white, nor the cube, nor the tart. What then is the salt? It is salt, pure and simple, but what is the truth of the salt? That it is what it is not. Hegel puts this point in more general terms: when we apprehend something, we take it as different from something else, especially ourselves, and so our taking (perception) is to take (perceive) something as the "opposite of itself." [39]

The language of perception differs from that of sense-certainty to the degree that perception itself differs from sense-certainty. The "this-here-now" of sense-certainty has become in perception a "this", taken together with its various properties, a "this-also-insofar as."[40] But, whereas in the former section we found that the language of sense-certainty misspeaks itself by meaning the particular while uttering the universal, here we find that the language of perception dies the death of a thousand qualifications. Instead of saying straight out that the thing is not a thing, that the salt is the opposite of itself, consciousness falls back upon the qualifiers, also and insofar as. This Hegel calls sophistry. Consciousness vainly wishes to simplify matters, to save itself from the inherent contradiction of perception (i.e., that a thing is what it is not). [41] The result is that:

> ...the truth which is supposed to be won by this logic of the perceptual process proves to be in one and the same respect the opposite... [42]

These words, this also and insofar as, prove themselves in the end to be empty. They are offered to ward off contradiction, but, as we will see, they lead consciousness to speak in tautologies. This is the subject of Hegel's next section on consciousness.

In the analysis of Force and Understanding, Hegel scrutinizes the language employed in the scientific explanation of objects by consciousness. Characteristic of this level of consciousness is the question, How? followed by a tautological answer.[43] Hegel's development of this theme borders on the mystical, so we might be better off taking a slightly different tack. Let me express in plain language what Hegel seems to have had in view.

Take the story of Sir Isaac Newton sitting under the apple tree. He is lost in his reveries when an apple falls to the ground. He asks himself, How? Not, How does an apple fall? but rather, How do terrestial bodies as such fall? Perhaps this prompts the further question, How do celestial bodies fall, or rather, not fall? One thing leads to another, and before he knows it, he has taken the apple's falling as due to the 'force of gravity' which is explicable in terms of the 'law of universal attraction'.

The force of gravity here is an example of what Hegel refers to when he says that the object of consciousness is Force. The object is not a thing, as in sense-certainty and perception. It is something altogether different, at once an "inner Thing" which lies beyond the things of sensation (the gravity 'behind' the apple) and the "laws of the Understanding" (universal attraction). Taken together these elements comprise Force as the movement by which the inner (gravity) is seen to be manifest outwardly (falling apple). Previously, this division appeared as the "contradiction" between perceived and perceiver, but here it is the coincidence of Force and Understanding.[44]

In fact, the inherent contradiction of perception has now become a reasonable distinction within consciousness. For the movement of Force, in Hegel's account, limns a syllogism in which the "inner Thing" and the "laws of the Understanding" are mediated by appearance.[45] To return briefly to the example of Newton's apple, gravity is the inner Thing, universal attraction is the Understanding, and the apple is appearance. But, Hegel's analysis exposes something peculiar in this syllogism. First, consciousness takes up with appearance. Then it supplies a law of the Understanding of which the appearance is said to be an instance. Finally Force is posited as the ground of the law. Thus appearance is apprehended as universal law, and universal law is explained as Force. However, Hegel maintains that this explanation is empty, as "*...Force is constituted exactly the same as law...*" [46] Let us return again to Newton's apple to illustrate this point. Consciousness begins with appearance, i.e., the apple. Next is supplied a law of the Understanding, namely, universal attraction. Then the force of gravity is invoked as the ground of universal attraction. Thus the appearance of the falling apple is said to be an instance of universal attraction, while universal attraction is said to be the understanding of the force gravity. Hegel remarks that, if the law of universal attraction says nothing more than that gravity is a force ,[47] the syllogism in question is a tautology. It explains nothing about the relation of the appearance (apple) and Force (gravity), having said all it has to say in expressing the relation of appearance (apple) and the Understanding (universal attraction). Thus, while the laws of the understanding account for appearance, they do so without saying anything meaningful about the inner Thing, about Force itself. The implication of this is that consciousness becomes trapped in the Understanding, and so comes to know nothing but itself. And yet, there is something fortuitous about this, for it is only then that consciousness becomes self-consciousness.[48]

Permit me to summarize. Consciousness asks how a given appearance is to be accounted for. The Understanding provides a universal law of which that given appearance is an instance. But consciousness cannot get beyond the realm of appearance and the laws provided it by the Understanding, and so it turns in upon itself, and becomes aware of itself as the movement of appearance and Understanding. Thereby it becomes self-consciousness. This truth is expressed in the tautology: I am I.[49]

To put Hegel's observation in slightly different terms, scientific explanation expresses the truth that consciousness comes to know itself in attempting to grasp its object in the world about it. Thus the language which articulates scientific laws is in an important respect tautological. But, what might be cause for uncertainty in scientific understanding is what Hegel deems the gateway to the "native realm of truth." [50] For, in leaving the world of sensation behind, consciousness has given up the quest for mere certainty, and has struck out instead for Absolute truth.

However, so long as self-consciousness remains subjective, that is, remains the relation of the subject to its limiting principles of understanding, it cannot bring itself to abandon the vain search for certainty in some thing outside of itself, and thus it does not grasp itself in its truth, its being.[51] The need for objective certainty leads self-consciousness out of itself and causes it again and again to fall into the trap of seeking objectivity in the realm of mere appearance. Only when self-consciousness comes finally to discover its appearance in another self-consciousness rather than in things, however, does it truly know itself.[52]

In Hegel's account, the 'I am I' of self-consciousness, or more properly the abstract 'I' of the Understanding, is changed by the presence of another into a 'We'. More simply put, we come to know ourselves only through others who know us. [53] This involves an important shift not in the terminology Hegel employs but in the meaning of existing terms. For, as he notes in this context, the 'I' is a 'We' and the 'We' is an 'I'.[54] Hegel's famous analysis of the master and the slave is an illustration of this basic point. But, as both parties are dependent in this situation upon one another, self-consciousness must, in Hegel's judgment, escape the struggle of master and slave. The principal reason for this is that dependent self-consciousness can only have a partial knowledge of itself; the other part is in the hands of the other. For the self to truly know itself, Hegel avers, it must be free. And such freedom is won by thinking, because thinking is, in Hegel's view, for the I to have itself --its whole and essential self-- for its object:

> In thinking I *am free*, because I am not in an *other*, but remain simply
> and solely in communion with myself...[55]

The freedom of self-consciousness, or thinking, passes through various forms before attaining its final end in the Unhappy Consciousness, a certain form of despair in which self-consciousness undoes itself, and yearns tragically for itself in the image of a unattainable, forever vanishing other.[56]

Hegel expresses this form of consciousness by again employing the language of syllogism. This time, however, the syllogism[57] in question is no mere tautology. It is rather the anticipation of Absolute Knowing, the goal of the phenomenology of mind and spirit. Just how this is the case is not readily apparent at this stage of Hegel's argument. What can be said initially, however, is that the discussion of the Unhappy Consciousness brings to an end a series of cycles through which consciousness has purportedly passed, and it marks the beginning of a new series of cycles. For from this point forward, we will see consciousness change from Reason, to Spirit, to Religion, to Absolute Knowing, and the insights won through the freedom of the Unhappy Consciousness, no matter how cryptic or dark, inform each of the several cycles.[58]

According to Hegel's analysis of self-consciousness, the middle term of this new syllogism unites the two extremes of universal and particular consciousness by rendering itself extinct. This middle term (Hegel calls it a mediator) is a self-sundering, and thus a fundamental, metamorphosis of consciousness. What more it is, is not clear. Unlike in all of his other analyses of the various stages or aspects of consciousness, here Hegel offers no examples or illustrations of his point. Some scholars have sought an allegorical interpretation for these passages by picking up on religious connotations of the terms employed.[59] I would not go so far as this, but would point out instead that perhaps the lack of illustration here is due in part to the fact that the notion of the Unhappy Consciousness, unlike the preceding descriptions of consciousness, is original with Hegel. There would, therefore, be no standard or traditional images or formulations to draw upon. Also, it should not be overlooked that Hegel depicts this stage of consciousness as an important transition in which examples and imagery must finally be replaced by more technical terms.[60]   Perhaps it is a shift from example to paradigm, where a general pattern is discerned in the parts, but no particular example can quite fully represent it. In any case, the language of self-consciousness transforms itself through the freedom of thinking into a new language, namely, that of Reason.[61]

In an important respect it is difficult to discern the differences between self-consciousness and Reason. Initially, at least, Reason articulates itself in the same 'I am I' structure as expresses self-consciousness. This is because, for Hegel, Reason is "thought thinking itself." But the all-important distinction between these two stages lies in the level of interpretation of the phrase. For, on the level of self-consciousness, 'I am I' connotes an unhappy situation in which consciousness must finally concede that, despite its desperate attempts to be certain in its knowledge of something outside of itself, it can only really know itself. But the 'I am I' of Reason goes beyond this, connoting a productive and fruitful recognition: for consciousness to know itself is for us to know everything, and this in a rigorously objective fashion. To utter 'I am I' in the voice of Reason is, in Hegel's way of putting it, to rediscover the *world*. Thus, while consciousness, in its narrowest sense, is the awareness of an object, and self-consciousness, in limited measure, is the awareness of oneself, Reason is the awareness that the self and its object are co-extensive in the form of the world. Just how Reason combines the objective and the subjective in the totality of the world, however, is not readily apparent. Hence Hegel is at great pains in the section on Reason to demonstrate that the self must abandon its object as such and see instead that 'I am the world'.[62]

At the stage of Reason, the syllogism of self-consciousness is expressed in the form of an infinite judgment.[63]   In general such a judgment conveys that something is what it is not by appealing to the mutual dependence of the terms in a given opposition. What strikes ordinary understanding as a bald-faced contradiction is presented here as the central truth of Reason. The Understanding heeds the principle of Identity. But Reason proposes that the essence of thinking is the "absolute difference between self-sameness and otherness." Thus, while it was problematic at the level of self-consciousness proper for the 'I' to discover that its 'other' was not an object, but rather a subjective structure of understanding, here the 'other' is known positively to be nothing but the 'I'. Or, to put it more succinctly, the 'I' includes difference within itself.

We recognize Hegel's point in our lived experience when we are separated from our known world. Whether this happens through the loss of loved ones, a dislocation from our home or work, illness, divorce, meditation, travel, adventures of all sorts, or our own death, we realize that most of the time our identity is spread around within the limits of our world. Our identity is distributed among our kith and kin, our concerns, possessions, and passions. We live largely 'outside' of ourselves. If we consider this insight in the abstract, we might express it as Hegel does: I am I as not I. And, to universalize this, we would say Reason attempts in all of its articulations to express that the self is what it is *and* all that it is not. This structure gives rise, in Hegel's estimation, to the "universal language" of the mores and laws of a people --to culture.[64]

Once consciousness finds its self in the real world, it has become Spirit.[65] Spirit speaks in the language of a people.[66] This is a living language, or language in the ordinary sense of the word. Note that in all that has preceded, Hegel has only drawn on certain aspects of ordinary language, but now we have before us full-blown, lived language. And, Hegel has provided this ordinary language with an extraordinary pardigm, namely, the unique syllogism of Reason. Thus language in general is seen to bespeak the infinite judgment whereby the self is known to be what it is not. As such, language takes on the status of being the determinate existence of our consciousness, the existential form of thinking called Spirit.[67] This process of self-alienation by which the self is found to belong to a community is what Hegel calls culture (*Bildung*).[68] Furthermore, the rupture of the self and its world in culture is the true subject of language.[69] Accordingly, one who can aptly express this rupture truly masters language, and bespeaks the development of Spirit in culture.[70] Thus the proper or "highest" form of language is distinguished neither according to the canons of formal logic, nor grammar, nor literary criticism. Much rather it is measured, at least provisionally, by the standard of a syllogism in which the subject (the self) and the predicate (the world) are comprehended in their complete incompatibility.[71]

The penultimate stage of Hegel's phenomenlogy is attained when the inherent rupture of self and world, which in its manifold forms constitutes culture, is transcended in the language of the "absolute unity" of consciousness and self-consciousness. The language which articulates this unity has various forms. All of them belong to culture, though each represent the possibility of overcoming culture through language. Thus they all participate in one capacity or another in the advance of Spirit toward finding its proper voice. And all alike belong to Religion.[72]

Religion, for Hegel, is the pure form of self-consciousness, beheld in an object. Religion and its object is distributed in his analysis among three basic types: natural religion, religion of art, and revealed religion. The first of these presents Spirit in the form of consciousness; consciousness beholds Spirit in the immediate shape of a natural object. The second represents spirit in the form of self-consciousness; self-consciousness creates Spirit in the shape of its own activity, i.e., as itself. The third is the unity of consciousness and self-consciousness; Spirit is revealed in the shape of the immediacy of self (self-consciousness) and the self as immediate (consciousness).[73]

Hegel considers each of these shapes of Spirit with regard to language. Natural religion represents a deficient (hieroglyphic) form of linguistic expression. The natural object is taken as a synthesis of the heterogenous forms of thought and the manifold of natural phenomena.[74] In the initial form of religion, a natural phenomenon is taken as the embodiment of Spirit. The highest form of such embodiment is that found in the likeness of an individual self-consciousness. Yet even here, the soul of the individual does not speak forth, but rather only expresses itself in deep, impenetrable wisdom.[75] Thus only the last two forms of religion have as their proper shapes some properly linguistic expression.

The first form of religion that is genuinely linguistic in kind, according to Hegel, is that of art. In its immediate form the language of the religion of art is the aesthetic representation of the divine in the oracle. Here the division of consciousness and its world is bridged in a deity that expresses itself in a language embodying the particular interests and national spirit of a people. This same language takes on a mediate form in the hymn. Here the deity is manifest solely in the language of a collective self-consciousness of Spirit. The linguistic arts of poetry, epic, and drama, however, represent, in Hegel's analysis, a grand attempt to join consciousness and the world in the form of divinity. For here the language of imaginative representation (*Vorstellung*) expresses fully universal humanity. Rooted in self-consciousness, this language is the soul existing as soul.[76]

Hegel conceives of epic as the expression of culture through the narrative representation of the acts of the gods. The determinate existence of epic, he notes, is language, and language which encompasses the universal content, or the completeness of the world. It is through the bard the the world is begotten and borne. The bard is compelled by the muse of memory, Mnemosyne, to give speech to the tension between mere mortals and the immortal gods. As expected, Hegel takes the universal song of epic as a syllogism which combines the universality of the gods and the individuality of the bard. The middle term of this syllogism is found in the heroes of the tale, who are individuals presented in the universal idea of the gods.[77] In sum, Hegel views epic as the necessary conflict of the gods and humans brought to speech.[78] The nature of this necessity is to prompt the emergence of a new form, what Hegel calls the "higher language" of tragedy.[79]

In tragedy it is the hero, not merely the bard, who speaks. The audience thus witnesses a self-conscious human being, enmeshed in the world through the assertion of will and right. The hero is portrayed in the first person by an actual, existing actor, who in his or her own words expresses the essential tie of particularity and universality visibly manifest in the mask.[80]

Hegel maintains it is only in comedy, however, that particularity and universality are fully commensurate. In tragedy the hero struggles to separate himself from a universal but alien fate, a fate put upon humans by the gods. Moreover, the actor must step out from behind the mask at the conclusion of the drama, separating himself from the fate of the hero.[81] In comedy, however, the actor projects a self-consciousness which is properly his, and that of the chorus and audience, and that of the gods themselves. The portrayal of self-consciousness in comedy, then, is the complete expression of universal consciousness in a particular person, rather than in the artistic abstraction known as an actor. Comedic self-consciousness is thus the self-consciousness of an individual, of universal selfhood in the form of a particular person.

Yet, being thus universal, the self-consciousness of comedy has an air of detachment from the play of particulars, displaying the irony that such universality should strive to assert itself on its own account as an individual.[82] Nevertheless, this self-certainty of the ironic consciousness of comedy is, according to Hegel, the sole repose of spirit.[83]

In the religion of art Hegel discovered that the necessary conflict of the gods and humans was suspended, for here divine being became the intrinsic limit of human being. The unity of the inward (universal) and the outward (particular) in the spiritual work of art took the form of the individual self-consciousness of the dramatic actor: I am I as not immortal. The drama of Spirit was thus manifest in the subject, in an individual self-consciousness.

This unity, however, is expressed from the side of the self, in the proposition, the self is the absolute being (*Wesen*). This phrase, therefore, does not belong to the sphere of religious language proper, Hegel maintains, because, while it captures the unity of self (self-consciousness) and world (consciousness), it does so in a one-sided fashion, from the perspective of the self. Or to put it slightly differently, the human self includes the gods as its ownmost limit. Thus the self-expression of the religion of art slips over into language characteristic of morality, an already superseded form of spirit. Hegel argues, then, that the religion of art belongs to the moral spirit.[84]

Hegel describes the regress of spirit from religion to morality expressed in the proposition, The self is the absolute being, as hapless. This latter form of spirit, the unhappy consciousness[85], is the tragic fate of a self that would be absolute. It is the counterpart and the completion of the repose of spirit expressed in comedic self-consciousness. For, comedic self-consciousness misspeaks itself in the assertion that the self is absolute being, that god is but the limit of human being, and thereby consigns itself to the fate of morality. In these words the tragic wins out over the comic, and the pose of spirit is shattered.[86]   The self is left with the feeling that the gods and humans share nothing in life.

By insisting upon its certainty in the judgment, I am All, the self makes itself subject, and absolute being, or substance, is made into a predicate.[87]   Thus, while the self is said to be substance, substance itself has been removed from the position of subject, and so has become a mere accident, predicated of the self. Accordingly Hegel maintains that the self has lost its substance in this assertion of its certainty. The judgment expressing the certainty of the self also expresses the loss of substance. Alone unto itself, bereaved of all essentiality, the self has lost even its self knowledge. The grief entailed transforms the judgment that the self is substance into the hard phrase: God is dead.[88]   Hegel portrays this grief at length in a moving passage:

> ... the ethical world and the religion of that world are submerged and lost in the comic consciousness, and the Unhappy Consciousness is the knowledge of this total loss .... Trust in the eternal laws of the gods has vanished, and the Oracles ... are dumb. The statues are now only stones from which the living soul has flown, just as the hymns are words from which belief has gone. The tables of the gods provide no spiritual food and drink, and in his games and festivals man no longer recovers the joyful consciousness of his unity with the divine. The works of the Muse now lack the power of the Spirit, for the Spirit has gained its certainty of itself from the crushing of gods and men. They have become what they are for us now--beautiful fruit already picked from the tree, which a friendly Fate has offered us, as a girl might set the fruit before us. It cannot give us the actual life in which they existed ...[89]

In revealed religion the imaginative representation of art is effaced. There is no longer such a separation between the self and god. The middle-term between the gods and humans is said to die.[90]   And the death of the middle-term, what Hegel calls the mediator[91], is the universalization of self-consciousness because it is the return of language into the self, into its concept.[92]

The effect of the death of the mediator is not complete in the sphere of religion. Indeed, Spirit cannot escape being imaginatively represented, so long as it belongs to religion.[93] The death of self-consciousness is still conceived of in language which articulates the death of the Mediator as the death of another.[94] Religion, in other words, remains art, and tragedy at that; art because it employs the language of imaginative representation proper to the narrative depiction of the absolute; tragedy because the story is about another.

The role of language in the final section of the *Phenomenology*, the famously incomplete statement of absolute knowing, is not apparent. Unlike the other sections of the work, this sketch of the consummate form of Spirit says nothing directly about language. It is, moreover, difficult to glean from it even implicit references to the role of language in absolute knowing. However, some conclusions might be drawn from the relation of religion and absolute knowing as it is presented there.

Hegel notes that in religion the content of absolute Spirit is given in the language of *another* self-consciousness. For example, the utterance, God is dead, when limited to the sphere of religion, is about another, namely, God, and not about me. In absolute knowing, on the other hand, that content is expressed in the language of the self: I=I.[95] This expression is no mere tautology, however, for it means that the self at once gathers itself (inwardly) from out of the world and empties itself out into the world. The language of absolute knowing is thus fully temporal, incorporating the casting and recasting of the self in the world. As Hegel puts it at the end of the work, the concept, as absolute knowing, is the inwardizing recollection (*Erinnerung*) and the Golgotha of absolute Spirit.[96]

The Speculative Sentence

Hegel's portrayal of absolute knowing in the *Phenomenology* suggests just enough about language to make it problematic. Manifestly the language of religion, from the hieroglyph of natural objects to the polished lines of the dramatic actor, is in some sense superseded in the comprehended concept. But is this to imply that language as such is superseded in the concept, or that the concept is the sole true form of language? To anticipate Hegel --and that is what must be done here-- one might venture that both of these implications follow: language finds its completion in being superseded by the speculative concept, and the concept, expressing the co-inherence of subject and substance, is the truth of language. But, if this is indeed the case, language must be so much a part of Spirit that it participates in its dialectic to the very last.

Once consciousness has gone through the various shapes outlined in the *Phenomenology*, it is prepared for the first time to grasp the philosophical import of language.[97] With a certain innocence, gained while sojourning in the strange regions of experience, consciousness overhears itself speaking in its mother tongue. And what it hears is extrordinary. Suddenly language is alive with the speculative power of the dialectic of Spirit. To speak is to bespeak the self and its world. Language, even when it purports to be philosophical, need not always fashion its discourse from propositions wrought in the mold of formal logic. Instead with language as its guide philosophy can begin to recognize and perhaps develop other patterns of discourse which, because they stem from constructions that have developed in the history of the language and its people, more adequately express human reason. Consciousness outstrips itself in a blossoming perspective.

What is finally discovered to consciousness in its language is the speculative knowledge, which, in comprehending the unity of opposites and the infinity of the positive and the negative, supersedes the categories and forms of traditional logic.[98] In the discussion of Hegel's *Logic* above it was seen how language encompasses both the categorical terms of traditional (Aristotelian) logic and the multivalent voice of speculative discourse. And our analysis of the *Phenomenology* indicated how consciousness can and must become aware of this truth. What must be added to this discussion is a brief examination of the root of speculative discourse. For Hegel's notion of a "speculative sentence" indicates how his original philosophy arises directly out of lived language.

The import of Hegel's development of the speculative sentence is manifold: it dismantles the dominant tradition of formal logic; it provides a means by which logic and metaphysics can be wed in a new speculative philosophy; it occasions a re-evaluation of the philosophical importance of ordinary language; it allows us to anticipate in ovo the course thinking will take once it becomes fully systematic.

Before analyzing these several aspects of the speculative sentence, let us pause to ruminate about the nature of the *Satz*. As with many of Hegel's key terms, this phrase has multiple meanings. In common usage, *Satz* denotes a jump or a leap, as in *einen Satz machen*. Just as commonly, however, it means "dregs" or "grounds." Among its more technical usages are "sentence" (grammatical) and "proposition" (logical). Let us begin with the latter two meanings.

Because the context of Hegel's phrase is philosophical in kind, and specifically logical, it is justifiable enough to take the *speculative Satz* as a proposition. But, when we recall that Hegel considered formal logic to be an abstraction from language, it becomes apparent that among this word's secondary denotations is "sentence." Thus, *Satz* indicates that logical propositions are still sentences belonging to ordinary language. Indeed, we realize that propositions are in the first instance expressions, no matter how formal.

This play on words is still more telling when one recognizes that, according to Hegel, a *Satz* is made up of a subject and a predicate.[99] For the subject and the predicate terms are at once logical and grammatical.[100] Moreover, the subject term, for Hegel, also denotes the philosophical notion of an individual consciousness[101], and so combines logic and grammar under the heading of self-consciousness.

The complex technical usages of *Satz* render its common meanings all the more suggestive in Hegel's phrase. For, a speculative sentence is surely in some sense a "leap" of thinking from out of the "dregs" of thought. Perhaps this seems strained. But, I do not think it is mere coincidence that in his Jena writings Hegel described speculative thinking as having a certain "magical" efficacy whereby reason rises Phoenix-fashion from out of the contradictory and antinomial ashes of the understanding to resplendent speculative brilliance. In fact the speculative spirit of language, as Hegel christens it, is the impetus by which language outstrips understanding through "coincidentally" expressing opposite meanings in the same word. Thus constructing a grand philosophical edifice on the shifting sands of ambiguity is indeed *einen Satz zu machen*! But, just such a revolution in thinking must be ventured if one is to grasp logic, grammar and consciousness in their linguistic unity.

Let us now turn to the first import of Hegel's speculative sentence mentioned above. In introducing the notion of a speculative sentence Hegel strives to overcome the limitations of understanding set down by the principles of formal logic. Such a logic rests upon a concept of identity (A=A) formulated in terms of the excluded middle and non-contradiction.[102] What must be accomplished for Hegel's task is the reinterpretation of this fundamental conception of identity according to the dialectic of spirit and in light of reason.[103] Here the leading insight is that identity does not mean that an individual is the individual, as in the so-called identical judgment of formal logic; it is not a mere tautology. Instead identity is the underlying unity by which something is said to be identical with what it is not, even with its opposite or contrary. This is to reconstrue the so-called infinite judgment of formal logic, which otherwise takes the subject and the predicate to be completely incompatible.[104] To state the matter in its complete form, Hegel grasps the identical judgment and the infinite judgment in their unity: I=I and ~I.

But just how is he able to reason in the face of such a bald-faced contradiction as is expressed in this logical formulation? His angle is to demonstrate that the content of thinking demands that it must assume this strange form. And the tour we took through the linguistic forms of the *Phenomenology* provided this demonstration, at least from the material side. What if we were to begin in the middle, as it were, where the form of thinking in general is taken along with its general content?[105] Or, to put it slightly differently, how would thinking speculatively express its sole, proper subject? Our answer is to be found in Hegel's discussion of God.

The subject which serves a paradigmatic role for Hegel's speculative sentence is "God."[106] This leads to certain implications for metaphysics and logic, as suggested by the second import of the speculative sentence mentioned above. The subject of a logical proposition such as "God is being" is, according to Hegel, not the Aristotelian substance which gains its attributes through predication.[107] It is much rather, a conscious subject whose essence is expressed (in whole or in part) in its predicates. Or, to put it in a more telling form, the subject-predicate structure of sentences is prior to and more encompassing than the metaphysical distinction between substance and accident.[108]

The originality of Hegel's construal of the relation of logic and metaphysics is nowhere more apparent than in his life-long interest in the so-called ontological proof for the existence of God. As early as *Glauben und Wissen* and as late as the lectures on the philosophy of religion, Hegel criticized Kant's famous demolition of this proof in the *Critique of Pure Reason*.[109] Kant's criticism, we learn, is telling only because he attacks the lesser form of the ontological proof, which conceives of existence as a predicate of God.[110] But, in Hegel's view, existence is the essence of God. Thus conceived, the ontological proof expresses the absolute unity of thinking (subject) and being (predicate), the foundation and coping-stone of true philosophy.[111]

When read speculatively the sentence, God is being, means that the subject has its meaning and existence in the predicate. This indicates the philosophical import of ordinary language. For, as was noted above, ordinary language comprises sentences which express the unity of predicate and subject in a way that is obscured by formal propositions. The obscurity of formal propositions is removed when we "re-read" the sentence as refering to the internal complexity of the subject, rather than as a straightforward attribution of a predicate to an already fixed subject.[112] Thus the ordinariness of the words, God is being (or, if you will, God exists), serves as the occasion for speculation to overturn formal reasoning. Furthermore, such words must be taken in the ordinary sense as belonging to a larger combination of words, or a context. Otherwise, their speculative gist will be erased through the abstracting and ossifying tendency of formal thought.[113]

However, if the truth of identity is made clear in the sentence, God is being, it is all the more fully manifest in certain other speculative sentences, specifically those in which is expressed the identity of subject and predicate, *despite* the fact that they are radically at odds.

The principles of excluded middle and non-contradiction are superseded in manifestly contradictory statements about God.[114] A sentence of particular interest here is: God is dead. When taken as a formal proposition, this sentence expresses a contradiction, God, being immortal and eternal, cannot reasonably be said to die. But, if taken speculatively, it bespeaks a basic truth of reason. For, as a speculative sentence, the words, God is dead, transcend and cancel the simple A=A of traditional understanding, and they do so in such a way as to call most urgently for further explication of the subject-predicate identity.

This brings us to the last import of the speculative sentence outlined above. The words, God is dead, are at first glance ordinary. Though the phrase may be shocking, still it employs only ordinary language. This is all the more apparent if we employ the self-same words as Hegel, for they are borrowed from a hymn[115]: *Gott selbst ist tot.* On the surface this sentence is a part of the traditional Christian confession. But, the critical reader will recognize that the term, *selbst*, renders the phrase problematic. The traditional confession attests to Christ's death, and not the death of God Himself. Thus this sentence seems to bespeak an atheistic truth. However, by returning to the phrase a third time, the speculative insight occurs that this sentence calls forth a new way of thinking, a unique way of conceiving the relation of subject and predicate which shares something both with Christianity and with atheism but which also outstrips either perspective. As such this sentence serves as a propaedeutic to a new system of thinking. It also provides the occasion of such a philosophy.[116]

Allow me to reflect briefly on the implications of this last point. The primary importance of grasping the speculative import of this and other such sentences about the divine being, according to Hegel, is to see that the languages of religion and philosophy share the same content. This saves philosophy from the fate of asserting that the abstract self alone is absolute reality, that the ethical sphere is higher than either that of religion or philosophy. Thus in effect Hegel steers philosophy away from atheism. The final importance, however, lies in establishing the properly philosophical understanding of religious language. For, if religious language is not put to the philosophical test, that is, if it is not rendered speculative, it tends to become entrenched in dogma and ossified. Traditional formulations of theology, because they belong to a creed which must either be accepted or denied, tend to obscure the speculative import of religious language for self-consciousness. Hegel has here in effect steered philosophy away from orthodox religion.

If Hegel assigns the formulations both of traditional theology and of traditional philosophy to a level below that of speculation, it is because he holds firmly to the superiority of speculative language for the critical and positive task of developing a true philosophy of spirit and reason. Thus Hegel's wish that philosophy should learn to speak German means ultimately that the absolute will be expressed in a speculative vernacular, as it were, which supposedly lies at the root of the German language:

> The absolute idea may in this respect be compared to the old man who utters the same creed as the child, but for whom it is pregnant with the significance of a life-time.[117]

Hegel describes this understanding of language in more properly theoretical terms:

> The philosophical proposition, being a proposition, gives rise to the opinion that the relation of subject and predicate and the procedure of knowledge are as usual. But the [speculative] philosophical content destroys this procedure and this opinion; one learns that what one supposed was not what one was supposed to suppose; and this correction of one's opinion requires knowledge to return to the sentence and reinterpret it.[118]

This last quotation brings up the final issue of language in Hegel to be considered here, namely, his style. Hegel is on all accounts difficult to read.[119] Some attribute this to a national penchant of German thinkers for the obscure. Others see in his style a richness and originality of expression without comparison. Still others aim between these extremes, accepting Hegel's supposition that his philosophy must be read at least twice.[120] If the last of these be chosen --and it seems to be the best option for one who would attempt to give Hegel his due, but no more-- the question arises as to the validity of Hegel's supposition. On what grounds may we claim that Hegel's philosophy warrants re-reading? Allow me to offer a suggestion.

Alexandre Kojeve's reading of Hegel, as was noted above, is rooted in the perspective that Hegel's language is the genuine representation of his system. Hegel's writing, he maintains, is the discourse comprising the system of his philosophy. In general I accept this thesis, but would limit it to the speculative element of Hegel's language. Hegel's writing is not the auto-effective speech of Absolute Spirit, nor is it the failed attempt to transcribe that speech. It is much rather the philosophical announcement of the possibility that thinking has a voice in which to speak that is not governed by formal logic. That voice of thinking is what Hegel called Absolute Spirit.

Hegel strove as a thinker and as a writer to emphasize a certain quality of language, that quality by which language forever says more than we intend. Double entendre, ambiguity, reflexive constructions; these and other elements of language determine that in speaking, consciousness expresses more than the simple sphere of its intentions. In this way language leads consciousness beyond itself to another, to a world of discourse and signification that can never be rendered the product of *my* consciousness.

Hegel saw deeply into the German language, descrying therein certain words and constructions that articulated a basic form of discourse. That discourse had been obscured, suppressed, or otherwise left unexploited by modern philosophy. Hegel took it upon himself to change all this. It is out of such language as holds within itself the identity and difference of thinking and being that Hegel's system arises. This has many forms in Hegel's philosophy, e.g., subject and substance;

subject and predicate; self-consciousness and consciousness; consciousness and world, etc, but in each of its forms is represented the limitation of formal reasoning as well as the possibility of overstepping that limitation through the aid of a new, discursive form of reasoning. That reasoning Hegel calls speculation, and he traces its course until he discovers its source and end in living language. He then begins to employ speculative discourse in the attempt to articulate the idea of philosophy, to found the system of philosophy. But his application and development of such discourse is only partial and preparatory. Hence we are left with an archaeological task: to exhume the remains of that incipient discourse. Let me contribute to this task by offering a brief summary of the relation between speculative discourse and traditional, formal reasoning.

Formal logic is an abstraction from language, designed to regulate speech, so that we express ourselves in well-wrought, logical propositions. Speech in this way becomes predominantly propositional. As such it comes to represent the basic expression of the understanding, the rules and principles of which are embodied in formal logic. The circle is thus complete: logic clarifies our speech; speech communicates propositions; propositions are the outward form of the understanding; the inward form is logic. But this elaborate tautology obscures the fact that formal logic is an abstraction, drawn from the repository of living language.

Hegel was moved to expose the fallacy of speech and formal logic. To this end he ventured that living language involves constructions which are not commensurate with formal logic. He focused upon the ambiguity and opposition inherent in many words and constructions. This quality of words he called the speculative spirit in language. With this as his wedge he set out to break the circle that had forged formal logic and language together. He attempted to return to language with a new innocence, an innocence gained through the perusal of the representative works of traditional reasoning. For in seeing the limitation of formal logic repeatedly instantiated throughout the history of Western thought and culture --in seeing that the understanding forever led from experience to paradoxes, and then to contradictions, to half-truths, to whole lies-- in seeing all this Hegel became, not weary and jaded, but infused with a new innocence for thinking. For in language, in that same language which he had spoken as a child with other children, he knew there was to be found a way of thinking that would not lead down the dead-end path of formal reasoning.

Thus speculative discourse is the reasonable product of a return to language. The aim is not to solve the problems of logic, but to sweep them aside as the by-products of over-ratiocination. By emphasizing certain elements of human language, speech and writing become a new affair. And, if one emphasizes those same elements of language as Hegel, the return to language marks the first step upon the path to philosophy as the system of speculative discourse.[121]

The paradigmatic example of Hegel's speculative discourse is the proposition, God is dead. For it is here, in this "hard phrase" --a paradox to philosophy and a stumbling block to religion-- that language most dramatically expresses the subversion of the governing rules of the relation of subject and predicate which have held since Aristotle. Here the predicate negates the subject, and yet it is only through this negation that the subject is known:

> Good Friday must be speculatively re-established in the whole truth
> and harshness of its Godforsakenness.

And once we realize that what is true of God is also true for us, we are prepared to speak conformably to the notion that self-knowledge is won only through self-negation, that to philosophize is to learn to die.

ENDNOTES

[1]GB p. 26. See also Hegel's thoroughly Kantian "Life of Jesus" in *Early Theological Writings*, trans., T.M. Knox (Chicago: University of Chicago Press, 1948).

[2]Logic, p. 34. From the preface to the First Edition.

[3]Ros. pp. 249-254.

[4]Just when Hegel "turned away" and under what circumstances will be addressed in the following chapter.

[5]Logic, Vol. 1, p. 54. The originality of Hegel's suggestion is encapsulated in his claim that logic possesses its own proper content, namely, thinking itself, and is not the mere collection of the formal rules of reasoning.

[6]Ibid. p. 62.

[7]Ibid. p. 42.

[8]Ibid. p. 42f.

[9]Ibid. p. 64.

[10]Ibid. p. 55f.

[11]This statement is much stronger in the original: *"Das Studium dieser Wissenschaft, der Aufenthalt und die Arbeit in diesem Schattenreich ist die absolute Bildung und Zucht des Bewusstseyns."* (SW, Vol. 4, p. 57)

[12]Logic, p. 69f.

[13]Ibid. p. 39f.

[14]Ibid. p. 42.

[15]See, for example, Hegel's early contributions to the *Critical Journal of Philosophy* in SW Vol. 1.

[16]Logic, p. 40.

[17]Ros. p. 9.

[18]Ibid. p. 10.

[19]The matter of Hegel's dislike of Latin stylists will be dealt with in detail in Chapter Three. Suffice it to say that he considered the coincidence of form and content in writing (that writing should bespeak its subject) to be more important than accepted, even classical style.

[20]Cited in Kaufmann, Hegel, p. 45f. Also Harris indicates that ambiguity had a wide-reaching role in Hegel's early thought, informing, for example, the important "paradoxical" conception of the necessary being of the Ideal:

> "But the tragic fate that produces all these distortions of life arises from the ambiguities implicit in the combination of the two propositions 'Being and union are synonymous' and 'That which is does not have to be believed.' We do not have to believe the simple truth. But it is an important part of the simple truth that we do have to have *some* ultimate belief in order to exist at all." (Night p. 13)

[21]Ros. p. 13. Again, this matter will be taken up in Chapter Three.
[22]Ibid. p. 16f.
[23]Though Hegel was ultimately successful in communicating his ideas, this did not come soon or easily. His early struggle with language is attested to in the following exchange between Goethe and Schiller:

> "Philosophy is not completely dumb, and our Dr. Hegel is supposed to have got many listeners who are not dissatisfied with his discourse." (Schiller to Goethe, Weimar, 9 November 1803. *Hegel in Berichten seiner Zeitgenossen*, ed. Günther Nicolin, Philosophische Bibliothek, Band 245 [Hamburg: Felix Meiner Verlag, 1970] p. 53)

> "I have spent very agreeable hours with Schelver, Hegel, and Fernow .... The thought has come to me regarding Hegel whether one could not do him a great service through technical training in speech. He is a thoroughly splendid person, but he is too much at odds with his expressions." (Goethe to Schiller, Jena, 27 November, 1803. Ibid. p. 54)

> "I see with pleasure that you are getting to know Hegel better. What he lacks could only be given him with considerable difficulty. Yet this lack of the gift of graphic representation is, in him, wholly the national fault of the Germans, and is compensated for --at least for a German listener-- through the German virtue of profundity and sincere earnestness.
> "I think that if you seek to bring Hegel and Fernow closer to one another it must be done through the one helping the other. In an intercourse with Fernow, Hegel would have to think about a systematic method in order to make his idealism understandable to him. And Fernow would have to abandon his superficiality. If you had both over to visit four or five times, and brought them into conversation, points of contact would certainly be found between them." (Schiller to Goethe, Weimar, 30 November, 1803. Ibid.)

> "I have already begun to put your suggestion to bring Fernow and Hegel together to work. Moreover, tomorrow afternoon I am going to have a tea party at which the most heterogenous elements will find themselves together..." (Goethe to Schiller, Jena, 2 December, 1803. Ibid.)

[24]Cited in Kaufmann, *Hegel*, p. 314.

[25]GW, Vol. 8, p. 354. Hans Kimmerle dates the *Reinschriftentwurf zum System der Sittlichkeit* in fall-winter of 1802/03.

[26]See the appendix to Hegel's *System of Ethical Life and First Philosophy of Spirit*, trans. Walter Cerf and H.S. Harris (Albany: SUNY Press, 1979) p. 185f.

[27]This is the thesis of Daniel J. Cook's *Language in the Philosophy of Hegel*. I will rely in large part upon Cook's work for our survey of the *Phenomenology*. But, because his analysis is sometimes incomplete or otherwise inadequate, I have supplemented his work with my own analyses of various segments of the *Phenomenology*.

[28]Hegel's term is *die sinnliche Bewusstseyn*.

[29]Hegel exploits the double-meaning of '*meinen*'. In terms of empirical consciousness, I 'mean' to say that the object is 'mine' in the sense that it is immediately present to me. However, Hegel plays with the word to show that what is 'meant' in language is not simply what I have in 'my' mind. Thus the meaning of my words supplants my possession of the object. In this way the phrases by which sense-certainty expresses itself undermine the claim that empirical consciousness possesses an object.

[30]PS p. 66.

[31]The affinity between common sense and ordinary language philosophy attests to this.

[32]Ibid. p. 58.

[33]Ibid. and also p. 60.

[34]Ibid. p. 62.

[35]Hegel describes this unity in the opening passages to the section on perception:

> "With the emergence of the principle, the two moments which in their appearing merely occur, also come into being: one being the movement of pointing-out or the *act of perceiving*, the other being the same movement as a simple event or the *object perceived*. In essence the object is the same as the movement: the movement is the unfolding and differentiation of the two moments, and the object is the apprehended togetherness of the moments." (PS p. 67)

[36]PS p. 72

[37]Ibid. p. 73.

[38]It should be noted that Hegel nowhere combines these terms in the way I have.

[39]PS p. 76.

[40]Hegel's description is as follows:

> "This abstract universal medium, which can be called simply 'thinghood' or 'pure essence', is nothing else than what Here and Now have proved themselves to be, viz. a *simple togetherness* of a plurality; but the many are, *in their determinateness*, simple universals themselves." (PS p. 68f.)

[41]The contradiction in question may require explanation. Hegel's notion of contradiction (*Widerspruche*) involves both a discord amongst claims made about a thing and a denial of the claim such language lays upon the thing itself. First, perception involves the 'contradiction' within the "plurality of reciprocally self-differentiating elements of a thing", that is, the cacophony, as it were, of propositions to name the determinate properties of the given thing.

This is less a contradiction, in the ordinary sense, than a colloquy of not necessarily opposite, but differing claims. Second is the 'contradiction' between what I have just described and the thing itself; the thing is not what may be said about it.

[42]Ibid. p. 77.

[43]That Hegel is indeed concerned with language is less apparent in this section than in the preceding. And the reference to the question, How? is in fact in the form of a warning not to raise the matter, or at least not to do so idly:

> "...we do not need to ask the question, still less to think that fretting over such a question is philosophy, or even that it is a question philosophy cannot answer, the question, viz. 'How, from this pure essence, does difference or otherness *issue forth* from it'?" (Ibid. p. 100)

Still, as is apparent from this quotation, Hegel addresses the need to know framed in this question.

[44]Ibid. p. 83.

[45]Ibid. p. 88.

[46]Ibid. p. 95.

[47]Though I have not provided his argument, Hegel does indeed make this claim.

[48]Ibid. p. 101

[49]Hegel's description of the matter is contained in the following passage:

> "But in point of fact self-consciousness is the reflection out of the being of the world of sense and perception, and is essentially the return from *otherness*. As self-consciousness, it is movement; but since what it distinguishes from itself is *only itself* as itself, the difference, as an otherness, is *immediately superseded* for it; the difference is not, and it (self-consciousness) is only the motionless tautology of: 'I am I'...." (Ibid. p. 105)

[50]Cook, op. cit., p. 55. Cook's discussion of language, which to this point has closely followed the structure of the *Phenomenology*, breaks off here and does not resume until the stage of consciousness Hegel calls spirit.

[51]Hegel's claim is that, so long as the difference between the I and itself does not take the form of being, it is not properly self-consciousness:

> "Hence otherness is for it in the form of a *being*, or as a *distinct moment*; but there is also for consciousness the unity of itself with this difference as a *second distinct moment*. With that first moment, self-consciousness is in the form of *consciousness*, and the whole expanse of the sensuous world is preserved for it, but at the same time only as connected with the second moment, the unity of self-consciousness with itself; and hence the sensuous world is for it an enduring existence which, however, is only *appearance*, or a difference which, *in itself*, is no difference." (PS p. 105)

[40]The following passage encapsulates the thought:

> "A self-consciousness exists for a *self-consciousness*. Only so is it in fact self-consciousness; for only in this way does the unity of itself in its otherness become explicit for it." (Ibid. p. 110)

53. Hegel's point is made briefly:

> "Self-consciousness exists in and for itself when, and by the fact that, it so exists for another; that is, it exists only in being acknowledged .... The detailed exposition of the Notion of this spiritual unity in its duplication will present us with the process of Recognition." (Ibid. p. 111)

[54]Ibid. p. 110.

[55]Ibid. p. 120.

[56]Ibid. p. 131f.

[57]Ibid. p. 136.

[58]Hegel gives a summary in the opening paragraphs of the section on Spirit which indicates the rehearsal of cycles I refer to. See ibid. p. 264f.

[59]See, for example, Findlay's attempt to develop a religious allegory in his commentary. Ibid.

[60]Ibid. p. 121f.

[61]Hegel states the matter in terms of the relation of being and acting, but it is to be noted that action, here, is an extension of thinking:

> "But in this object, in which it finds that its own action and being, as being that of this *particular* consciousness, are being and action *in themselves*, there has arisen for consciousness the idea of *Reason*, of the certainty that, in its particular individuality, is has being absolutely *in itself*, or is all reality." (Ibid. p. 138)

[62]See, for example, p. 139f:

> "Now that self-consciousness is Reason, its hitherto negative relation to otherness turns round into a positive relation. ...Apprehending itself in this way, it is as if the world had for it only now come into being ....for the existence of the world becomes for self-consciousness its own *truth* and *presence*; it is certain of experiencing only itself therein."

[63]Hegel's reference is fairly inconspicuous, as it comes in a later passage of the work. The basic point is that consciousness expresses itself in a proposition which cancels itself. This proposition is an infinite judgment: *das <u>unendliche Urtheil</u>, dass das Selbst ein Ding ist, -- eine Urtheil, das sich selbst aufhebt.* (PG p. 269) An infinite judgment is to be distinguished from an affirmative or a negative judgment. An affirmative judgment takes the form: S is P. A negative judgment takes this form: S is not P. An infinite judgment takes the form: S is non-P. It would seem that Hegel renders the syllogism of self-consciousness as an infinite judgment:

I am I.

I am not I.

I am I as not I.

[64]I have passed over the section on Observing Reason in order to pick up the theme of language at its next stage. In the subsequent section, on the Actualization of Self-consciousness, Hegel considers the substance of self-consciousness as it is articulated in custom. Ibid. p. 213.

[65]Hegel's point is clear:

> "Reason is Spirit when its certainty of being all reality has been raised to truth, and it is conscious of itself as its own world, and of the world as itself." (Ibid. p. 263)

I will skip over the discussions of the "ethical world" and "morality" which frame the section on culture. For, in keeping with the language of Reason formulated in the syllogism, culture is the middle-term which unites the ethical world and morality in their difference. As such, culture can be isolated as the true embodiment of the language of Reason. See ibid. p. 411f.

[66]We may now resume our summary of Cook's work, but we will intersperse his comments in the framework of the present discussion of the infinite judgment. Cook notes the following about the role of language in Spirit:

> "Through speaking, consciousness transcends its own isolated existence and realizes that its experiences are not arbitrary or unique, but part of a larger community or ethos. Language is the first and most immediate existential form of intersubjectivity." (Cook, op. cit., p. 78)

Though Cook emphasizes the problem of intersubjectivity here, still his portrayal conveys Hegel's more far reaching conviction that the language of existential reality bespeaks the syllogism of Reason.

[67]It should be noted that this is the first instance in Hegel's analysis in which language resembles what we would ordinariy recognize by this term. In the preceding sections, he focussed only on certain aspects or constructions of ordinary language. Now it is the full-blown language of a culture which Hegel has in view.

[68]Cook's view of the role of language is especially apt here:

> "Language represents the external embodiment (Dasein) of ego itself. Individual consciousness finds in the act of speaking a way of adequately projecting itself into the world." (Ibid. p. 85)

The key phrase here, however, is "adequately", for only in language are the self and its world united in thinking.

[69]Cook notes that language, for Hegel, is tied inextricably to culture:

> "Language embodies, more than anything else, this ruptured state between consciousness as subject and the world about it." (Ibid. p. 89)

[70]Cook expands upon this basic point:

> "By exposing the contradictory or dialectical nature of thought and reality itself, the individual in culture, through its rupturing outlook and expression, performs an essential role in the spiritual development of human consciousness." (Ibid. p. 90)

[71]I suspect that Cook skipped over the section on Reason in the *Phenomenology* because that on Spirit better suits his somewhat one-sided presentation of Hegel's notion of language. But, as I

have indicated, it should not be overlooked that Hegel establishes the proper form of language-
-and especially language as the expression of the rift which is culture--to be the infinite judgment,
or the self-transcending assertion of consciousness.

[72]The transition from culture to religion in the *Phenomenology* is not easy to grasp. To anticipate,
it involves the transformation of the infinite judgment of culture, namely I am I as not I, into the
infinite judgment of religion, namely, God is dead. The total incompatibility of God and death
represents and is the dramatic unfolding of self-consciousness. Essential here is the fact that in
religion consciousness becomes a fully linguistic reality for the first time.

[73]As in the preceding discussion of spirit, it will be seen that the two forms of religion which
frame the middle-term, religion of art, are mediated by it. Thus art emerges as the true language
of religion. Accordingly it is taken up again in the final section of the *Phenomenology*, on
absolute knowing.

[74]PS p. 424.

[75]Ibid. p. 423f.

[76]Hegel makes his point in terms of the particularization and universality of subjectivity:

> "...the complete separation into independent selves is at the same time the
> fluidity and the universally communicated unity of the many selves; language
> is the soul existing as soul." (Ibid. p. 430)

[77]Ibid. p. 441.

[78]The following passage refers to the gods:

> "They are the universal, and the positive, over against the *individual self* of
> mortals which cannot hold out against their might..." (Ibid. p. 443)

The syllogism in question seems to be something like the following:

All gods are immortal.
<u>Heroes are not gods.</u>
Heroes are not immortal.

The point is that the conflict of the gods and humans depicted in epic revolves around the issue
of mortality.

[79]Hegel gives the language of tragedy the following place:

> "This higher language, that of Tragedy, gathers closer together the dispersed
> moments of the inner essential world and the world of action: the substance
> of the divine, in accordance with the nature of the Notion, sunders itself into
> its shapes, and their movement is likewise in conformity with the Notion. In
> regard to form, the language ceases to be narrative because it enters into the
> content, just as the content ceases to be one that is imaginatively presented.
> The hero is himself the speaker, and the performance displays to the audience-
> -who are also spectators--self-conscious human beings who know their rights
> and purposes, the power and the will of their specific nature and know how to
> assert them." (Ibid. p. 443f.)

[80]Ibid. p. 444. The point hinges on the fact of utterance. The hero here utters his fate for himself. The conflict of the gods and the humans is no longer expressed in indirect discourse, as in epic. The syllogism expressing this would perhaps run as follows:

All gods are immortal.
I am no god.
I am not immortal.

As an example of this, consider Hamlet's parting words, "I am dead, Horatio .... Horatio, I am dead."

[81]Thus the matter involves, not only the choice of direct discourse over indirect discourse, but also the choice of truly self-expressive direct discourse over a masked, or seeming, self-expression.

[82]Ibid. p. 450. The syllogism that would express this is perhaps something like the following:

All gods are immortal.
Humans are not gods.
Humans are not immortal.

It will become clear from what follows that the feeling of ease, gained by expressing the fact of mortality in the abstract, is but a fleeting and ultimately illusory moment.

[83]Ibid. p. 452f. But, as will be seen, this moment of repose leads seamlessly into the pit of an empty self.

[84]Ibid. p. 453f.

[85]Ibid. p. 454.

[86]The following passage presents Hegel's conclusion in stark terms:

> "We see that this Unhappy Consciousness constitutes the counterpart and the completion of the comic consciousness that is perfectly happy within itself. Into the latter, all divine being returns, or is the complete *alienation of substance.* The Unhappy Consciousness, on the other hand, is, conversely, the tragic fate of the certainty of self that aims to be absolute. It is the consciousness of the loss of all *essential* being in this *certainty of itself*, and of the loss even of this knowledge about itself--the loss of substance as well as of the Self, it is the grief which expresses itself in the hard saying that 'God is dead'." (Ibid. p. 454f.)

[87]The point is difficult. Apparently, in expressing the judgment, I am All, the self determines that the divine belongs to the human only in so far as it represents the negative limit of the self: I am All *as* non-divine. Thus the conception of the self is limited by what it is not, namely, the divine, and the divine is likewise made into a mere limit.

[88]Again we have a difficult notion. The infinite judgment of culture, I am I *as* not I, is transposed into the following proposition: I am I *as* 'God is dead'. That is, I am I only in so far as I am not the god named in the utterance, God is dead.

[89]Ibid. p. 455.

[90]At this point I can only speculate about Hegel's thinking. It would seem that our syllogism would run as follows:

All gods are immortal.
I am not a god.
I die.

Here the middle term between the gods and humans is the positive act of death, expressed in the judgment, I die. In Hegel's way of speaking, the middle term itself is said to die.

[91]The significance of Hegel's term, Mediator, requires some explanation. His development of this notion is tied to his analysis of the revealed religion. In this religion, ostensibly identifiable with certain elements of the Christian religion, God is said to become man, and die. Thus death is the unity of God and man. It is as such the middle term of the syllogism in question, as it is the mediator between God and man. As mediator between God and man, death unites the death of a given person with the death of God, so that death in each case comes to signify the end of dying alone (as a person), and the end of the abstraction named in saying that God is dead. Hence the death of the Mediator is not my death, nor is it the death of God. Yet, in saying, I die, it becomes the meaning both of my death and the death of God.

[92]Hegel describes the passing away of artistic expression as follows:

> "The immediately preceding element of picture-thinking is, therefore, here explicitly set aside, or it has returned into the Self, into its Notion; what was in the former merely in the element of being has become a Subject." (Ibid. p. 475)

The implication of this seems to be that the words, I die, are the return of language into its concept.

[93]Ibid. p. 479.

The implication seems to be that the syllogism of the revealed religion would run as follows.

God became human.
All humans die.
God is dead.

Here the infinite judgment of self-consciousness is expressed indirectly, about an other. But because this judgment is about subject and substance as such, it expresses the last thing that can be uttered in the language of self-consciousness before that language undergoes the radical transformation into speculative discourse.

[94]Ibid. p. 477.

[95]Ibid. p. 489.

[96]The sentence is somewhat famous in secondary literature:

> "Their preservation, regarded from the side of their free existence appearing in the form of contingency, is History; but regarded from the side of their [philosophically] comprehended organization, it is the Science of Knowing in the sphere of appearance: the two together, comprehended History, form alike the inwardizing and the Calvary of absolute Spirit, the actuality, truth, and certainty of his throne, without which he would be lifeless and alone.

Only from the chalice of this realm of spirits foams forth for Him his own infinitude." (Ibid. p. 493)

[97]Cook, op. cit., p. 137.

[98]Ibid. p. 138f.

[99]Hegel puts this in a slightly different way when he extols the philosophical virtues of German. His native language, he maintains, is superior in its manifestation of thought in nouns and verbs. (See Logic, p. 39f.) Grammatically speaking, the noun is the subject and the verb the predicate.

[100]See Stephen Houlgate, *Hegel, Nietzsche and the Criticism of Metaphysics*, p. 142f. Houlgate make this point in reverse, emphasizing that not all grammatical constructions are logical. Clearly, he recognizes that some are.

[101]See Jere Paul Surber, "Hegel's Speculative Sentence", p. 214f.

[102]Cook avers that Hegel:

"... attacks the basic laws of two-valued formal logic - i.e., the Laws of Identity, Excluded Middle and Contradiction - with a view to realizing his primary philosophical objective: the promotion of dialectical reason through an awareness of the limitations of the ordinary, static 'either-or' judgments of understanding." (Cook, op. cit., p. 143)

[103]I distinguish between spirit and reason here because, in regard to language, the former is the phenomenal while the latter is the eternal aspect of language, or *logos*. The distinction is implicit in the following passage by H.S. Harris:

"Hegel recognized the independence of 'Phenomenology' because he saw that this question about critical and speculative Reason must be asked about 'Spirit' and 'Reason' (the phenomenal and the eternal aspects of the Logos respectively) and not about 'Logic' proper (as the science of the *eternal* Logos)." (Night p. 417)

[104]Cook, op. cit., p. 143. See also Houlgate, op. cit., p. 146.

[105]Houlgate points out that the speculative sentence must be universal in scope, and not merely a particular expression of some state of affairs. See op. cit., p. 146.

[106]This is a rather controversial claim. There is much in Hegel's philosophy to suggest its truth, but there is perhaps as much which undermines it. Cook, for his part, supports the claim (op. cit., p. 145). Surber too worries this question, but with a different result. He maintains that Hegel's choice of example is indeed the most general speculative sentence possible. However, he also adds that there must be a "common form" of all such sentences (op. cit., p. 216f.) Houlgate appears to follow Surber's lead, but he goes so far as to exclude Hegel's example from the list of genuine speculative sentences. His reason is that "God" is a representational word, and therefore is not, striclty speaking, a universal concept. I would add that Hegel's choice of example is crucial just because it is problematic: he begins here because "God" is the absolute, paradigmatic subject.

[107]See Surber, op. cit., p. 214.

[108]Ibid.

[109]See CPR pp. 500-507.

[110]See, for example, SW, Vol. 1 p. 314.

[111]In the essay on common sense in the *Critical Journal of Philosophy* Hegel describes his early interest in God as a subject of philosophy as the attempt to:

> "... once again place God absolutely at the apex of philosophy as the sole ground of all, as the unrivaled *principium essendi* and *cognoscendi*." (Ibid. p. 199)

Even if Hegel no longer refers to God in this capacity in his later philosophy, still the unity of thinking and being represented by the ontological proof holds center-stage throughout Hegel's thought.

[112]See Houlgate, op. cit., p. 148. Cook, Surber and Houlgate are all to be credited for pointing out that speculation advances not through presenting new concepts or propositions cut from whole cloth, but rather through reconstruing the ordinary meaning of the sentences involved. It is not inappropriate to call this process re-reading, as we will soon see that Hegel himself uses such an expression. It might also be noted that the famous Hegelian term, *Erinnerung*, connotes just such re-reading, a re-membering which is also an inwardizing, or intensification of meaning. This matter will be dealt with in more detail in Chapter Three of the present study. See also PS p. 39.

[113]Houlgate, op. cit., p. 149. Houlgate rightly emphasizes that a speculative sentence cannot stand on its own. For, simply stated, if it did, it would either be a word, refering to some other thing, rather than a structure of reference inherent to the subject, or it would be what Hegel calls the "bare bones" of logic. Surber comes close to making this mistake when he identifies the subject-predicate relation as the "most elementary form of language" (op. cit., p. 213). But he does go on to say that the very complexity of this relation gives rise to *further articulations*. Both Houlgate and Surber thus identify the speculative sentence as the kernel from which the Hegelian system emerges as discourse.

[114]Cook puts it as follows:

> "The realm of Spirit as Spirit is reached only when the laws of Identity and Contradiction are aufgehoben. This can best be seen in the meaningfulness of apparently contradictory statements about God or Absolute Spirit: contradiction itself is a manifestation of the Absolute." (*Op. cit.*, p. 150)

It might be noted in passing that the speculative sentence, God is dead, anticipates the speculative sentence, I die, for the identity of subject and predicate expressed in the former is essential to grasping the identity expressed in the latter. As it is with God, so too is it with me.

[115]I am not sure what to make of this, but aside from the grammatical and logical usages of *Satz* is the technical musical meaning: a *Satz* is a musical phrase made up of at least three notes.

[116]The most remarkable contribution Surber makes to this topic is just this. He notes that the speculative sentence, because it is an ordinary utterance of language, provides a non-philosophical avenue to philosophy. He, however, makes no mention of the phrase, Gott selbst ist tot. But see Hegel's comment regarding this occasion in the preface to the *Phenomenology* (PS p. 44).

[117]From the *Logic*. Cited in Cook, op. cit., p. 160f.

[118]From the *Phenomenology*. Cited ibid. p. 166f.

[119]I have been told that Mark Twain once quipped that Hegel's writings are the closest thing we have to chloroform on paper.

[120]Cook ends his work with a brief summary of the various opinions to be found regarding Hegel's style. His own opinion is non-committal:

> "Hegel's philosophical terminology is grounded upon his conception of philosophizing and the validity of this conception alone can serve as the justification for the language he used to express it." (Ibid. p. 174)

[121]In an independent study I have compared Hegel's linguistic innovations regarding logic with Heidegger's grammatical innovations regarding ontology. That study is presently an unpublished manuscript entitled, "Hegel, Heidegger and the Grammar of German Philosophy."

2 | LIFE

In the last chapter we saw how the phrase, God is dead, limns the paradigm of a transformative philosophical language, namely, speculative discourse. That discourse lies at the heart of the Hegelian philosophy, providing the vehicle for a thinking set loose from the constraints and antinomies of formal reasoning. In this chapter I will present the biographical context of Hegel's first utterance of the death of God in 1802. The focus of attention will be Hegel's move to Jena in 1801. For this move was perhaps the most important event in his career. It was there in the midst of Goethe, Schiller, Schelling, the Schlegel brothers and many others that Hegel came into his own as a thinker. Most important, in my judgment, was the effort he expended on the issue of language. In Jena he became aware of the limits of his own verbal abilities as well as the general restrictions imposed on thinking by traditional religious and philosophical terminology. He liberated himself from the dead bones of dogmatic and formal language and taught himself to speak in paradigms. He was forced to let his close friend Hölderlin go, for the young poetic genius had slipped into irreversible madness while they lived together in Frankfurt (1796-1801).[1] Then Hegel's father died (1799). But in Jena, it was God Himself who was said to have died (1802).

To anticipate, we will see how Hegel's utterance of the death of God in 1802 is coeval with his coming of age as a philosopher. Thus the death of God will not be approached as the product of a mature philosopher, but rather as the occasion for maturity. In taking up this profound thought, in bringing it to speech, Hegel came under its influence. So much so that it shaped his entire vocation as a thinker.

To put matters thus is to suppose the utterance of the death of God marks a change in Hegel. One might ask, then, who Hegel was before 1802 and who he became thereafter. And indeed recent commentaries attempt to identify a significant transformation in the man on or about the turn of the century. However, it is not apparent what role the utterance of the death of God plays in all of this. In what follows I will attempt to make that role clear.

This period has drawn considerable attention in the secondary literature. It is generally recognized that Hegel's thinking underwent significant changes about the time he moved to Jena. But this has not always been the case. Hegel's contemporaries thought of him at that time as riding on the coattails of the brilliant young Schelling. With the benefit of hindsight, however, this perception has gradually given way. Now Hegel is widely considered to be Schelling's better. Indeed, it seems that Hegel's greatness as a thinker began to take shape when he was abandoned in Jena by his one time friend.

Some of the more obvious factors drawing attention to this period are that Hegel took his first post as a university professor during this time; he published his first works then; he appears at that time to have shifted his manifest interest from religion and history to philosophy. Less obvious, though no less important, factors center around questions of Hegel's intentions in moving to the "literary glut" in Jena, his growing concern with the need to develop a system, and his developing interest in language.

Prevailing scholarship does not identify the the death of God as a major factor in Hegel's development. There are two principal reasons for this. First, Hegel's earliest and arguably best biographer, Karl Rosenkranz, presented the view that Hegel was a born systematic philosopher. From his point of view, everything written during the Jena period (including the utterance of the death of God) appears to be nothing more than Hegel's attempt to render his system in language understandable to his students. Accordingly, we are led to seek the origin of the Hegelian system, and with it his philosophical coming of age, in the earlier Bern and Frankfurt periods. Attention is thereby drawn away from the first years at Jena. Second, H.S. Harris, disputing Rosenkranz's dating of certain crucial writings, has successfully argued that the Hegelian system is apparent no earlier than 1800, and that even then it appeared in an immature form. Harris's account is that before the turn of the century Hegel aspired to be a religious reformer, but that he soon gave up his designs on a new folk mythology for a post as a professional philosopher.

These two prevailing views are misleading to a certain degree. On one hand, Hegel was not born with a system in mind, and any reliance on this notion leads one to overlook the innovations of the Jena period. Harris has called our attention to the relevance of the Jena writings, and so has gone a long way towards counteracting Rosenkranz's hagiographical fallacy. Yet, Harris goes too far in his suggestion that Hegel's references to the subject of religion after 1800 (including the death of God in 1802) are all throwbacks to the language of faith and a failed ideal. For the implication is that Hegel's use of religious language does not have a philosophical import.

Both Rosenkranz and Harris are correct, however, in emphasizing the role of language in the Jena period. Hegel did not merely translate his system into a more popular language when he accepted a job in philosophy at Jena. Before this he had neither a philosophical language nor a system to call his own. Nor did Hegel merely trade the language of faith in on the language of reason. Instead he discerned the makings of a genuine philosophical discourse within a fundamental religious confession, namely, God is dead. This phrase provides the paradigm of a transformative philosophical language. This new speculative discourse announces Hegel's coming of age as a thinker, for it constitutes the living kernel of his philosophical system.

During his stay in Jena, Hegel worked under the assumption that thinking is a matter of seeing that the imagistic language of religion has its root in a living vernacular which itself supersedes the language of formal reasoning. Thus language as such becomes thematic, taking precedent over traditional religious and philosophical formulations, and providing the grounds for their criticism.

It should be clear now that Rosenkranz was correct in identifying Hegel's tendency to "popularize" his language, but incorrect in drawing the conclusion that Hegel had a system prior to this turn toward ordinary language. Before he discovered the speculative value of his mother tongue, all he had was the fragments of other thinkers' systems. Harris too is correct in part, for Hegel did abandon the popular language of religion in favor of techinical philosophical terminology, but not because he had at last given up the misguided desire to be a religious reformer, and chose instead to become a professional philosopher. Rather he perceived that thinking, if it was to be rigorously philosophical, had to take its departure from religious language. Philosophy had to dip into the well of living cultural (especially religious) language so that it could displace the stultifying terms of traditional reasoning. This was to render a speculative system from out of the fruits of living discourse. By its very nature, however, this task would involve a reformulation of traditional religious language (as well as language in general), for such would have to undergo a certain philosophical initiation. Hegel addresses both sides of this matter in the following passages. First is his concern with avoiding obscure philosophical terminology:

> Yet that which is in itself must not have this strangeness for us and we must not give to it this strange aspect through a strange terminology. Much rather we must consider ourselves convinced that Spirit itself lives everywhere and that it expresses its forms in our immediate popular

language. They occur in ordinary talk, mixed and muffled in sonorous concrete statements ...[2]

Second is the quite different affair of developing a more appropriate language for philosophy:

> To be sure, it is necessary for us to take refuge in strange terminology, if we do not find the determinations of a concept present in our language. It is not unusual for us to do violence to language and to construct new forms out of old words.[3]

We can see here the twofold task which faced Hegel in his attempt to address the philosophical problems and promise of language. First, he sought to discard the foreign (especially Latin) terminology of traditional philosophy in favor of his mother tongue. Second, when his mother tongue was not up to the task, he would exploit it to develop genuinely new philosophical expressions. This project became the turning point in a new life of the mind. The fulcrum was the "ordinary" saying, God is dead.

Let us now turn to the details, to consider more closely the nature of the watershed which developed in Hegel's years in Jena. The immediate problem at hand is to determine the value of the preceding period in Hegel's career, namely, the Frankfurt period.

Three main issues bear upon this concern. First, certain fragmentary writings stemming from this period have been presented as the earliest form of Hegel's systematic thinking. Second, much has been made of a supposed crisis Hegel suffered during this period, although dispute surrounds the nature and the severity of this development. Third, reference is sometimes made to an intellectual conversion of Hegel during the Frankfurt years. Let us first turn our attention to the matter of Hegel's Frankfurt writings.

The Frankfurt documents vary considerably in subject matter. Hegel composed pieces in many genres--everthing from mystical theology, to historical criticism, to geometry, to poetry, to politics, to astronomy and more. Moreover these diverse documents have come down to us in various ways, some being preserved by the author, others by friends and associates, while still others have been lost except to the memory of those who once saw them. Consideration of these writings is further complicated by certain mistakes which, once committed, have been repeated through the years. Thus arguments still rage over the proper dating of certain pieces. Sometimes their very authorship is called into question. Whether all of the confusion associated with this period is warranted or not remains to be seen. Hegel's close collaboration with Hölderlin during this period, for example, certainly gives one reason to look at these documents with a critical eye. Also, Hegel was in the habit of copying extensive excerpts from what he was reading, whether it be the morning paper or Kant's philosophical treatises. To a certain extent, this further muddies the water. And, because the manuscripts from this period are fragmentary and undated and even sometimes secondhand, things can be very treacherous indeed.

But in all fairness it should be added that intellectual historians are sometimes prone to make more of certain documents than is justifiable. In the case of someone as broadbased and difficult to read as Hegel, it is tempting to seek out lesser writings to cast light on the greater whole. Whatever the reasons, however, the Frankfurt period is a veritable quagmire. Accordingly, opinions about the status of the period as a whole are diverse. Various accounts depict Hegel as shifting his attention during this period from theology to politics[4], from popular religion to philosophy[5], from philosophy to "speculative pneumatology"[6], etc. Let us leave aside the larger issue for now and concentrate on the status of certain key documents.

Rosenkranz dated two important manuscripts as belonging to the Frankfurt period. They became known in the literature as *Logik, Metaphysik, Naturphilosophie* and *System der Sittlichkeit*. Niether were ever published, nor were they complete, even in Rosenkranz's time. However, because they are both relevant to the question of system, they have become the object of much scrutiny. Rosenkranz maintained that these manuscripts represent the oldest, most original form of the Hegelian system.[7] This claim remains viable, but it is now accepted that Hegel wrote these documents while he was in Jena.[8] Thus, if these do indeed represent the earliest form of Hegel's system, we must conclude that the genesis of the system post-dates the Frankfurt period. But this further complicates the matter.

Aside from the disputed manuscripts mentioned above, Rosenkranz identified Hegel's system in another document. He thought it was comtemporaneous with the other two, but only because he had been mistaken about the dating of *Logik, Metaphysik, Naturphilosophie* and *System der Sittlichkeit*. Now known as the *Systemfragment*[9], this document represented to Rosenkranz an application of Hegel's system to the concept of religion. That the *Systemfragment* belongs to the Frankfurt period has not been questioned, as the manuscript displays the date, 14 September 1800, at its conclusion. However, that the fragment represents Hegel's system, even in outline form, has been seriously challenged. Knox has argued that, while it may have certain elements in common with Hegel's system, there is no reason to view it as more than an essay in theology.[10] Olson even accepts that the piece may well have been written by Hölderlin.[11]

H.S. Harris[12], however, has found reason to see more in this essay than do others. Knox's opinion is based on what is now extant of the fragment. But this is a mere fraction of what Rosenkranz had before him in the early 19th century. Harris accepts that the present *Systemfragment* is but the conclusion of a much longer document which has been lost. He thus ventures that the *Systemfragment*[13] belongs to a larger system which began to emerge in Hegel's thinking during the Frankfurt period.[14]

Harris is not alone in emphasizing the significance of this early period for the development of Hegel's system. Georg Biedermann seeks the origin of Hegel's system in the Frankfurt documents as well as in writings stemming from the still earlier Bern period.[15] Here emphasis is put on the importance of a unpublished essay entitled *The Positivity of the Christian Religion*. The focus of Biedermann's attention is the "dialectical" character of this essay. Supposedly it presents a new and uniquely Hegelian conception of religion in which contradiction is the primary element. Biedermann takes this as the germ of a system devoted to accounting for the totality of social transformations. His is a worthwhile observation because it indicates Hegel's long-standing preoccupation with contradiction as a cultural form, but we must be wary of placing such a premium on the socio-political aspect of Hegel's thought during this period lest we overlook his contributions to the life of the mind.

This early period remains one of interest not only because of the writings Hegel composed then, but also because of important events in his personal life. Some have pointed to these events to provide circumstantial evidence for their interpretations of Hegel's writings. This is the second issue listed above as having a bearing on the Frankfurt period.

Biographical details are marshalled from Hegel's stay in Bern and Frankfurt which would reflect the probable state of mind of one who was to embark upon such a serious endeavor as compiling a system of philosophy. Biedermann, for his part, depicts Hegel in this period as a seriously disillusioned youth, ready for a new start. Hegel had been an enthusiastic supporter of the French Revolution, but its manifest failure shook him deeply:

> ... Hegel's inability to conceive of [the failure of the Revolution] from the philosophical position of Kant (and Fichte) or to overcome it religiously brought him to protracted, psychological depression, to hypochondria. He sought to take action against the incipient spiritual crisis through labor which mounted to the limits of psychological capacities.[16]

Biedermann's dramatic portrayal compels one to find deep significance in the resulting fragmentary writings of this period. But it should not be omitted that, however dramatic this crisis might have become, Biedermann describes it as building over a long period, from the summer of 1796 in Bern through the following years in Frankfurt. Only gradually was it transformed into a newer and more mature perspective in the autumn of 1800.[17]

The so-called "crisis of Frankfurt" became an item of interest because it provided a dramatic setting for the emerging genius of the "system." Rosenkranz mentions it only in passing, however. And, it is clear from his account that Hegel's gloominess preceded his move to Bern:

> In the fall of 1796 Hegel traveled from Bern straight away to Stuttgart to see his family again. On the strength of his sister's account, he was quite introverted, almost gloomy, and only in quite close circles did he thaw out to the cheerfulness, which one had earlier found in him.[18]

A slight account of the event might be expected of a work spare of biographical details, such as Rosenkranz's. But he goes a long way in dispelling any suspicion that Hegel was unhappy once he arrived in Frankfurt. He enjoyed a certain leisure for his thinking, a most pleasing social atmosphere, and the close friendship of Hölderlin and others. No mention is made of brooding over political concerns which might have followed Hegel on his move from Bern.[19] This is not to say that he would not have reason to grieve in his new residence. Eventually he would have to come to grips with Hölderlin's collapse into madness. But this is quite another matter.

Harris plays down the psychological aspects of the affair, suggesting that Hegel's 'crisis' was probably no more than the sort of failure of confidence we all sometimes feel.[20] Yet he still maintains that because of the *Systemfragment* the period is a watershed in Hegel's development.[21] This "lost essay" represents, in Harris's judgment, a religious intuition that was to be transformed into a philosophical system in Jena, specifically, that which Rosenkranz mistakenly thought belonged to the Frankfurt period, i.e. *Logik, Metaphysik, Naturphilosophie* and *System der Sittlichkeit.* Harris describes the significance of this document as follows:

> It is no surprise to find that at Jena the religious-aesthetic intuition that we meet here, first becomes a theoretical or intellectual intuition, and then develops into the discursive mode of expression that typifies Hegel's later systematic works. When he wrote the *Systemfragment* Hegel had already decided to become a professional philosopher if he could.[22]

It should be noted, however, that there is "no surprise" in finding this transformation, only if one has already assumed that Hegel had decided to become a "professional philosopher." But, is it not just this transformation from religious-aesthetic intuition to discursive system which makes the philosopher, not the will of the would-be philosopher which explains the transformation? Indeed, as we shall see, the very crux of the matter is how what Harris calls intellectual or theoretical intuition enables art and religion to gain philosophical import.

This is to bring up the third matter which bears on the Frankfurt period, namely, Hegel's supposed intellectual conversion. While Harris prefers to speak of Hegel's decision to become a philosopher, others have ventured that Hegel underwent an intellectual conversion while in Frankfurt. Olson, for example, has provided a detailed argument that Hegel converted from a "dialectic of renunciation" represented by Hölderlin and the Greek Ideal to a "dialectic of transcendence".[23] This latter represents Hegel's turn toward Christianity and the promise of christological conceptions of transcendence for philosophy. But this emphasis of the relation of Hegel and Hölderlin distorts the whole of Hegel's development. This is nowhere more apparent than in the inappropriateness of Olson's romanticized label. Conversion is too strong a notion for what may have happened in Frankfurt. Indeed the language of conversion seems to be a rhetorical play used or implied by those who would read Hegel's mature philosophy as a gloss on the Christian faith. Whereas Harris and others may be guilty of a certain "psychological" fallacy in interpreting Hegel's development, Olson is representative of an even more distracting "pneumatological" fallacy.

Let us take a moment to review. It is generally agreed that the most important event in Hegel's development as a systematic thinker was his move to Jena. It was here that he first began to teach at the university level; here that he first published his writings; here too that he made the aquaintance of some of Europe's greatest intellectual figures; here that he finished the final pages of his greatest work, the *Phenomenology*, just as the Emperor Napolean rode into town. Nevertheless some have focused attention on the Frankfurt period, arguing in effect that Hegel's systematic bags were packed before he left for Jena. The importance of the Jena period is undercut by the presence of the *Systemfragment* of 1800 and the circumstances of its composition. This document was written during Hegel's last days in Frankfurt, while he had begun to witness the tragic demise of his closest friend, and just after the death of his father. Romantic tendencies are perhaps behind the notion that the "Frankfurt crisis" was the symptom of great inspiration, but the idea is somewhat appealing. Naturally enough, we would value highly anything written while Hegel was so inspired. We might see such writings alternately as the last gasp of a passing, though passionate, enthusiasm or as the first sign of an impending explosion of insight. But the most cogent account of the matter is that provided by Harris. Hegel, it seems, was not debilitated by any crisis, whether caused by something which he had suffered or by intense anticipation, but rather found the confidence as well as the occasion to leave Frankfurt and all that it represented behind. He was led on by a new and compelling ideal, to become a philosopher. Thus the watershed year becomes 1800, when the young thinker formed the resolve to move to Jena.

But, as we will soon see, Harris's rendition draws more on the invisible cause of Hegel's latent intention to philosophize than on the manifest evidence of an emerging system. In fine, Harris's account is too much about the man's mind and too little about his writing. And if this is true of Harris, it is all the more true of Biedermann.

If language has the import in Hegel's philosophy that I think it does, the tendency to explain Hegel's writings by appealing to the mystery of his mind is mistaken. It is not the mind, in Hegel's philosophy, which carries thought, but the word.

Let us further investigate the pitfalls of trying to conjure Hegel's spirit. Rosenkranz stolidly maintained that the man's life was marked throughout by a singleness of mind and a steadiness of character to match. He makes no mention of Hegel's supposed psychological crisis in Frankfurt. At the same time he places the earliest sketches of Hegel's system so far back ('90s) as to draw attention away from the efforts of the philosopher some years later in Jena. In fine Rosenkranz paints a picture of Hegel as one who was throughout his life destined to be a pedagogue of systematic philosophy[24]:

> The greatest difficulty of my work lay in the peculiarity of Hegel's essence to have steadily developed itself gradually from all sides scientifically. His production was a tranquil procession of his intelligence, a continual working out of his entire person. Accordingly, his biography lacks the charm of the great contrasts of passionate leaps, and averts total monotony only through the thorough significance of its hero.[25]

> The history of a philosopher is the *history of his thought*, the history of the formation of his system.[26]

There is genuine truth to Rosenkranz's perspective. As is apparent from even a cursory examination of his writings, Hegel was a person who never changed his mind, save to expand it yet more in comprehending something else. Thus even his day-journal, written while he was in the Gymnasium at Stuttgart, will strike the student of Hegel's mature thought as no less than uncanny. The presence of ideas, methods and phrases in his earliest writings are premonitory of the mature thinker's habits and concerns.

Nevertheless, as almost everyone but Kant, Hegel moved about a good deal during the course of his life, making new friends and enemies, taking up various jobs and residences. That such incidental changes were more than superficial to Hegel's life is manifest in the enthusiasm with which he threw himself into new situations. This enthusiasm is evident throughout Hegel's early correspondence. He writes to Schelling in 1794, for example, and expresses his good fortune in having left Tübingen behind for the greener pastures of Bern, even as he wishes for still another environment:

> I long very much for a situation --not in Tübingen-- where I could bring to fruition what I formerly let slip by, and could even on occasion set my hand to work. I am not completely idle, but my occupation, heterogenous and often interrupted as it often is, does not allow me to achieve anything proper. [27]

His letter of 1800 to Schelling is still more enthusiastic about the prospects of a move from Frankfurt to the fertile ground of Jena. [28]

If it is too much to say that he was everywhere at home with himself, it is true that wherever Hegel was, he engaged himself deeply in the affairs and reality of his surroundings. J.N. Findlay remarks how Hegel's stay in Bern as a tutor was somewhat uncomfortable.[29] Despite his unhappiness, however, Hegel devoted himself to a detailed study of the emergent historical reality of his place of tenure. And, in keeping with the spirit of Bern, he even began to compose in French.[30]

It might seem somewhat self-serving of one who has undertaken to write on Hegel to claim that in this person is to be found a genuine union of constancy and alteration; he has come down to us as the philosopher *par excellence* of continuity in change, identity in difference. However, if one notes the degree to which Hegel and his intellectual and aristocratic contemporaries of the late eighteenth century strove to make themselves great and imposing personalities of classical life, it is perhaps not an overstatement to say that Hegel self-consciously modeled himself after the eternal, the everlasting, the timeless ideal of humanity. Hans-Georg Gadamer describes this pervasive ideal of humanity in the following words:

> Herder, more than anyone, transcended the perfectionism of the enlightenment with his new ideal of 'reaching up to humanity', and thus prepared the ground for the growth of the historical sciences of the nineteenth century. The idea of self-formation or cultivation (Begriff der Bildung), which became supremely important at the time, was perhaps the greatest idea of the eighteenth century ...[31]

This idea of the interrelatedness of the development of the self and of the sciences was, in Rosenkranz's judgment, not wasted upon Hegel. He remarks upon the notion of culture which Hegel helped to formulate:

> Culture means nothing but thinking and determination of the will through thoughts, through laying hold of the universality and necessity of the universe in its unity. Philosophers will always rise from the dead. There can never be a last system of philosophy.[32]

The essential connection of thought and reality, self and world, expressed here came to permeate the age. But initially it was discernible only in the details. For example, Hegel's journals and letters, as also those of his kindred spirits of the age, are composed in private, but written for the view of like personages. The task of being a person involved in large part the presentation of oneself to that society, real or ideal; present, future or past, by which one most sincerely wished to be measured. This opposition of self and world was the essential principle held in common by Hegel and Goethe.[33] And, based on the extent to which each accomplished a reconciliation of this opposition in philosophy and poetry, respectively, one might judge Hegel and Goethe to be the leading world-figures of this epoch in German culture.[34]

Those who found the true measure of humanity only in what is classical, timeless, and great conducted and expressed themselves as though they were worthy of thus being judged. Even if sometimes they did this in what might strike us as a rather mediocre fashion, in the age of Storm and Stress, the dilettante towers above the expert and crass technicians of industry and execution. In the paradigmatic cases of Hegel and Goethe, it was not only the mastery of their individual fields of philosophy and poetry that draws the attention of posterity, but also and more importantly that both were very serious, if amateur, scientists. Thus their spirit of broad experience provides the true compliment to their achievements in literature. And, if an age can be measured by what it imagined, suggested, hoped and intended, rather than merely by what it had time and energy to execute, the late eighteenth century of European culture will strike us as rich indeed.[35]

Hegel, being both child and parent to this culture, ventured to loosen the bonds of habit and dogmatism, to change, but to change by way of embracing the manifold experiences of life in their eternal verity. He was perhaps, as H.S. Harris rhapsodizes "a real, live Wilhelm Meister."[36] Or we might go so far as to follow Walter Kaufmann in his suggestion that Hegel might have quoted Goethe's *Faust* as a motto for his concept of experience:

> And what is portioned out to all mankind,
> I shall enjoy deep in myself, contain
> Within my spirit summit and abyss,
> Pile on my breast their agony and bliss,
> And thus let my own self grow into theirs, unfettered ... [37]

Thus Hegel's restlessness, as that of the times generally, can be viewed as a sign of the recourse of the eternal ideal of humanity in the world of culture.

The name which German speakers gave to this recourse, *Bildung*, connoted, not the simple addition of something new to what was already in place, but much rather a placing of the new in such a way as to point back to the universal origin and timeless aim of life itself. Hegel and his contemporaries strove, somewhat paradoxically it might seem, to place the coping-stone atop the arch of culture, so that it was also at once the corner-stone and foundation of life.

If the above portrayal of Hegel's times is true to life, Rosenkranz's description of the thinker's nature misses at least in part. The opposition of self and world, learning and life, is not likely to have been deeply felt by one who thought the problem of culture could be solved merely by presenting one's system of philosophy. But such a one Hegel was not. For, as even Rosenkranz remembers against his own thesis, Hegel did not always aspire to a system of philosophy.[38]

Once Hegel had developed a systematic philosophy, according to Rosenkranz, he was fully committed to working it out in detail, and presenting it to his students and colleagues. Thus, through the course of his career, he came to see the final necessity of presenting this system in his own words. In Berlin Hegel is supposed to have "gradually got used to the notion that for speculative education salvation could indeed be found only within his philosophy." [39] Yet this was not the young Hegel.

In contrast to Rosenkranz, H.S. Harris weaves a compelling tale of the young Hegel's vocation as a *Volkserzieher.* Rather than a proponent of the scientific systematization of philosophy, Hegel is portrayed as a reformer, one who would liberate the German people from the bonds of tyrannical Christian culture by reviving the spirit of Greek religion through the practical efficacy of a new mythology.[40] But, according to Harris, around the turn of the century Hegel paused. Napoleon had been victorious in France, and it seemed that Hegel was forced to give up on his ideal, for the window of opportunity had passed.[41] Hegel, "convinced that his work was not after all of any practical use", laid down his pen, and took stock of his vocation. Hegel now came to realize, in Harris's judgment, that he must become a philosopher, and expertly so.[42] Thus Hegel abandoned the project of a new mythology, and set to work in earnest to establish a rigorous system of scientific knowledge.

At this point Harris's thesis is in accord with Rosenkranz's, for, rather than a religious-aesthetic ideal, the German people were now seen to be in need of a serious philosophical education.[43] To thus construe Hegel's abandonment of the ideal of a folk mythology in favor of an academic career draws renewed attention to the issue of pedagogy and its role in understanding the development of the thinker's early period. For Hegel's turn toward academics involves not only his new role as a professor at Jena, but also his experiences as a student at the Stuttgart Gymnasium. A consideration of these experiences should shed some light on his role in Jena.

The two principal accounts again come from Rosenkranz and Harris. They are in agreement that Hegel's early education was informed by the principles of the Enlightenment, but that the curriculum was drawn from classical antiquity.[44] Harris adds that 'Enlightenment' must here be understood as an extension of Renaissance humanism, and that therefore the overriding concern was to face the question 'What use is all your historical and literary erudition to the progress of the human race?' This question, Harris maintains, is the point of departure for Hegel's independent studies.[45]

Harris and Rosenkranz paint a composite picture of Hegel as a very critical student. And both connect this with the student's fervent interest in living history rather than in the dead forms of past knowledge.[46] And, as we will see in the next chapter, this critical attitude developed during the Jena period into his unique reading of the history of philosophy. But beyond his critical attitude, Rosenkranz and Harris give us accounts of the young Hegel with little in common. Rosenkranz depicts a brilliant but somewhat eccentric student, given to contradictions, strange phrases, unusual style[47], and genuine pedantic zeal.[48] But this obsession with arranging the substance of his learning was, in Rosenkranz's opinion, testimony to Hegel's commitment to systematic thought.[49] Harris, in his turn, portrays this student as an aspiring educational reformer who only gradually became interested in the broader, philosophical question of human nature.[50]

The emphasis upon Hegel's ideas in Rosenkranz and his ideals in Harris is representative of the general differences between these two portrayals. And while the contrast between Rosenkranz's and Harris's portrayals of Hegel while in the Gymnasium might seem slight, once they have worked their influence upon the treatment of later periods of Hegel's career, these initial characterizations become important indeed. Most particularly, at the beginning of the Jena period, the question becomes whether Hegel has turned back to philosophy after a sojourn in folk religion or whether he has turned to philosophy for the first time.

Hegel's turn to academia, as recounted by Harris, coincides with what Rosenkranz refers to as the "didactic modification" of Hegel's system. Rosenkranz describes this as follows:

> In Jena Hegel had at first presented his system in the complete abruptness of its original conception, but a few years experience with this sufficed to make it apparent that such a form might not suit an academic lecture. He had to vitally perceive the need for a more *popular* presentation. The cleft was too great between the profound spirit that developed itself with audacious abstraction in this system and the consciousness his students brought directly with them to lecture.[51]

As we have seen above, the system to which Rosenkranz here refers was not yet written. Indeed, what Rosenkranz took to be merely a "popular" presentation of the system is now generally recognized as the first form of Hegel's systematic philosophy.[52] Thus we cannot meaningfully speak of a modification of any system here. However, what we do find in Rosenkranz's account of the "didactic modification" is that the development of Hegel's system may well be coeval with his concern for pedagogy. And it is in this respect that Findlay refers to the development of Hegel's dialectic in this period. For "philosophy, as the *Science of Reason* - by the universal manner of its being - is, by its very nature, for *everyone.*"[54] And so the emergence of the system in the classroom merges with Hegel's attempt (considered in the previous chapter) to teach philosophy to speak German. An analysis of the role of language in the Jena lectures will reveal the relation between the Hegelian system and the German people, between learning and life, in the thinker's own words and personality.

Rosenkranz's treatment of this material is somewhat familiar by now: Hegel felt the need to make his idea more accessible to his students by downplaying the use of technical philosophical terminology. Rosenkranz mentions several important aspects incorporated into Hegel's introductory lectures dealing with the system in its totality:

> Now Hegel worked over the philosophy of *nature* and of *spirit* into comprehensible presentations, as he no longer made the dialectical element stick out so formalistically, but rather allowed it to blend more with the matter. He abandoned the formal ideality, with which he had previously accompanied the logical side of the presentation step by step, laid down the major determinations more categorically, and strove in the execution for a, so to speak, *genre-painting-like* illustration, which often extended into a critique of the times, not merely in a scientific, but also in a political and religious respect.[55]

These apparent modifications were accompanied by several suggestions as to the proper form of philosophical discourse. The first mentioned by Rosenkranz has to do with terminology:

> Moreover [the introductory comments] yielded important utterances about terminology in general, namely, to execute it, so far as possible, entirely in the mother tongue.[57]

He elaborates this point by quoting from Hegel's lecture manuscript:

> Our thought is not yet properly at home in our language; it does not control language, as it should be, but rather we foster blind reverence for what is customary.[58]

That Rosenkranz describes this fundamental philosophical challenge as a didactic modification reflects his conviction that Hegel's primary concern in these lectures was to bring his system down to the level of his students. For Rosenkranz speaks of the "need of philosophy" (which we will examine in our next chapter) as an academic expedient.[59]   To construe matters in this way presents the so-called modification of the system as the philosopher's condescension to the sphere of the public.

Harris gives a different account of the matter. Indeed he argues for an almost diametrically opposed position in which Hegel strives to become a fully philosophical *Volkserzieher*: the task is to express the ideal of the people in a conceptual form drawn out of the German language.[60] Rather than focusing upon the distinction between the philosopher's language and that of the student, as does Rosenkranz, Harris draws attention to the philosophical efficacy of the mother tongue:

> ... Hegel wants to insist at the outset that the conceptual comprehension of the most ordinary expressions of everyday life contains all the riches of religious experience; and it does not refer us to a beyond, but shows us how our present life can be understood as self-sufficient.[61]

If Harris and Rosenkranz are in agreement that the issue of language is crucial in the Jena period, they differ fundamentally as to the implications of this. Based on the two portrayals we have reviewed of Hegel up till his time in Jena, we might venture to accept Harris's depiction of the young Hegel as a *Volkserzieher* and Rosenkranz's portrayal of Hegel as a teacher of systematic philosophy, with respect to the mature thinker. For, the "didactic modification of the system" is no modification at all, but the emergence of the system for the first time. As is manifest by the role of language in the Jena lectures, the *Volkserzieher* has to become rigorously philosophical in his use of language, and in so doing he becomes a self-modeled philosopher of the German people. Thus the issue of language as such emerges as the medium through which the young Hegel becomes mature. To anticipate, Hegel's maturity is formulated in 1802 in the language of the death of God.

Let us again pause to review our findings. The advantages of choosing Harris's account of the young Hegel are clear. Rosenkranz's work is commendable in the respect that it puts Hegel's thought first. This properly philosophical biography includes glosses and passages of material which is now lost. It is thus still important to one who would see the outlines of Hegel's entire corpus of written work. But the flaw of the work, beyond its mistaken dating of certain manuscripts and the origin of the system, is that it presents the entirety of Hegel's writings as amendments to a system of philosophy. The career of this thinker thus becomes a monotonous unfolding of his supposed system, as we saw Rosenkranz admit above. From whence did Hegel's thinking originate? In the end I suspect here a certain christological fallacy whereby Hegel's writings are seen as the outpouring of a pre-incarnate Logos. But more on that later.

Harris's work, solidly grounded in the latest chronologies and informed by a truly impressive knowledge of Hegel's thought, corrects the distortions of Rosenkranz's study by focusing upon Hegel's development as a thinker, rather than upon the presentation of his system as such. And, because Hegel apparently aspired at different times to be a scholar, a reformer, a philosopher, Harris provides a view of the fissures in the development of the young thinker. With these to punctuate the flow of the writings, it becomes a more discrete, if not simpler, task to sort out when and why Hegel wrote what he did.

The principal disadvantage of Harris's account, however, is that it too rigidly applies the question of vocation to Hegel's writings. By suggesting that Hegel was now a scholar, now a reformer, now a philosopher, Harris means to read Hegel's writings in light of their author's likely aims and purposes. However, Hegel had the habit throughout his life of copying extensive excerpts out of everything from the morning paper to Kant's *Critique of Pure Reason*.[62] He also worked seriously on various translations of both classical and modern texts.[63] Moreover, Hegel was not wont to reflect upon his vocation. Much rather he was generally occupied by the related but significantly different concerns of how to make a living, what he would read and write next, and where an with whom he would reside. If we can trust his own words, he did not move to Jena to become a philosopher, but to renew his friendship with Schelling:

I have watched your great public career with admiration and joy; you leave me the choice of either speaking humbly of it or wanting to display myself before you as well. I avail myself of the middle term: I hope we rediscover each other as friends. ...no matter how long it takes I must also know how to honor fate and must wait upon its favor to determine how we will meet.[64]

With these important factors in mind, it begins to look as though the question of Hegel's vocation is too narrow to understand his early period.[65] The changes from scholar, to reformer, to academic philosopher proposed by Harris seem to stem from a twentieth-century conception of the intellectual life in which the competing needs of scholarly publication and teaching are met by offering courses drawn from one's speciality. But Hegel did not seem to become a hostage of the university in this way. As a professor he possessed the freedom and the initiative to teach subjects in which he was and was not expertly trained.[66] As he moved through subjects in university courses (and later at the Gymnasium at Nürnberg) he relentlessly strove to express the whole. This preoccupation with the totality of learning and life was charateristic of Hegel throughout his adult life, but nowhere more so than in the period here in question.

If we accept Harris's depiction of the young Hegel as a *Volkserzieher* and Rosenkranz's portrait of the mature systematic philosopher, the principal question of this enquiry remains unanswered. To put it baldly, one would still wonder whether the utterance of the death of God by Hegel in 1802 ought to be taken as the last-ditch effort of the *Volkserzieher* or a new beginning for the systematic philosopher. If taken in the former sense, the death of God could conceivably belong to the mythology of a new folk religion which rejected Christian theism and its other-worldly attitude toward affairs of the people and its nation. On the other hand, if taken in the latter sense, one might well expect that Hegel's new philosophical system was designed to strip scientific knowledge of all reliance upon the images and myths of God, the afterlife, and the like. Rosenkranz and Harris are not silent on this matter however.

For his part, Rosenkranz takes Hegel's philosophy as inherently bound to religion.[67] Moreover, he maintains that Hegel's philosophy is Protestant in character:

I deem Protestantism that form of religion which grounds the reconciliation of God and humankind through certitude, so that the essence of human self-consciousness has as its content the divine self-consciousness and thus has freedom as its form.[68]

The freedom of self-consciousness is, according to Rosenkranz, expressed both philosophically and religiously in the death of God. Harris accepts Rosenkranz's view, and elaborates it:

> The existence of man in the world is a 'speculative' Good Friday ....
> The 'speculative' Easter [69] must come from man's own triumph in the effort to 'know himself.'[70]

The question thus becomes one of deciding whether the death of God belongs to religion or to philosophy, or perhaps to a new 'philosophical religion.'

Harris is apparently undecided on this matter. The indecision comes about in the following way. Harris considers the *System of Ethical Life* (1802/03) to point backward to the project of the *Volkserzieher*, where religion is the absolute form of experience, and forward to the *First Philosophy of Spirit* (1803/04), where philosophy takes top honors.[71] Thus the *System of Ethical Life* appears as the watershed in Hegel's development, providing the systematic transition from religion to philosophy. However, Harris further associates the *System of Ethical Life* with the introductory lectures on philosophy (*Logic and Metaphysics*) and the *Differenzschrift*, both of which belong to the year 1801. Harris in effect pushes the watershed back to 1801.[72] He thereby creates a lacuna between these writings and the *First Philosophy of Spirit* of 1803/04. And the entire project of the *Critical Journal of Philosophy* of 1802/03 and its reference to the death of God falls within the bounds of this gap. Consequently Hegel's utterance of the death of God (composed prior to June in 1802) would come after the 'philosophical' turn of mind, but before any outward manifestations of such a turn. But what, then, are we to make of Hegel's utterance? Is it a throwback to the former religious ideal, a last word by the disheartened *Volkserzieher*? Is it rather a premonition of the philosophy to come, a first principle of all scientific thinking? I don't think these questions can be answered within the framework of Harris's study.

Perhaps a more insightful approach to the connection between the thinker's life and the death of God can be found in Hegel's emergent intellectual personality, informed by the critical and speculative writings of this period, especially those dating from 1801-03.[73] The question I would like to pose is, How does the utterance of the death of God compel a thinker first to criticize religion and then to go beyond it in the form of speculative philosophy? In the chapter to follow we will see how Hegel developed the notion of speculative philosophy. The matters of criticism and interpretation will become paramount in our attempt to grasp the utterance of the death of God as the paradigmatic expression of a new kind of thinking and of a new career in the life of the mind. The occasion for this turn in the history of thought is what Hegel calls the "need of philosophy."

ENDNOTES

[1]A fine account of the matter is presented in Alan Olson's *Hegel and the Spirit* (New Jersey: Princeton University Press, 1992) p. 84 *passim*.

[2]Karl Rosenkranz, *Georg Wilhelm Friedrich Hegels Leben*, p. 183.

[3]Ros. p. 184.

[4]See, for example, Franz Wiedemann, *Hegel*, trans. Joachim Neugroschel (New York: Pegasus, 1968) p. 132.

[5]We will investigate Harris's claim to this effect.

[6]See Olson, *Hegel and the Spirit*, p. 12.

[7]Ros. p. 183.

[8]See H. Kimmerle's chronological appendix in GW Vol. 8, p. 348.

[9]For the entire document see T. M. Knox, *Early Theological Writings*, pp. 309-319.

[10]Ibid. p. 309, footnote 1.

[11]See *op. cit.* p. 85. Olson includes a brief discussion of this dispute as presented in the works of Dieter Heinrich and Otto Pöggler.

[12]See Sunlight.

[13]Harris agrees with modern scholars in assigning the other manuscripts to the Jena period. See, Harris and Knox, *Hegel's System of Ethical Life and First Philosophy of Spirit*, p. 3. Though he does not expressly mention the manuscript on *Metaphysik...*, Harris surely accepts the present dating of this work in the Jena period. For the dating see *Dokumente zu Hegels Entwicklung*, ed. Johannes Hoffmeister (Stuttgart-Bad Canstatt: Frommann-Holzboog, 1974) p. 474.

[14]Harris's views will be developed in more detail in the following discussion.

[15]GB p. 33.

[16]Ibid. I have provided the translation of this and the passages to follow.

[17]Ibid. pp. 28-32.

[18]Ros. p. 80. I have provided this and the translation to follow.

[19]Ibid. p. 81.

[20]Sunlight p. 265.

[21]Ibid. p. xxxii.

[22]Ibid. p. xxxii.

[23]*Op. cit.* See especially Chapter Four.

[24]Ros. p. 4.

[25]Ibid. p. xv-xvi. Rosenkranz is not alone in his retrospect that a great potential lie with the infant born in Stuttgart in August of 1770. Take, for example, the sentiment of the opening lines of Biedermann's biography:

> Stuttgart, 1770. The August sun brooded heavily over the long-respected capital of the province of Württemburg, picturesquely surrounded by the forested heights of the Neckartals. Nothing hinted at a particular event. Life in the city went its usual busy way. And, if not many years later, the name of one of its sons would become famous throughout all of Germany, hardly anyone would have called to mind this day in 1770. (GB p. 7)

[26]Ibid. p. 21.

[27]See *Hegel: The Letters*, trans. Clark Butler and Christiane Seiler (Bloomington: Indiana University Press, 1984) p. 28. The last phrase of this passage could also be translated "...does not permit me to come into my own." The difference is not great, though it does emphasize Hegel's concern at the time to achieve not just anything, but to develop his own thought.

[28]Ibid. p. 64.

[29]J.N. Findlay, *Hegel: A Re-Examination* (New York: The Macmillan Company, 1958) p. 29.

[30]Ros. p. 61f.

[31]Hans Georg Gadamer, *Truth and Method* (New York: Crossroads Press, 1975) p. 10.

[32]Ros. p. xxi.

[33]Karl Löwith, *From Hegel to Nietzsche; The Revolution in Nineteenth-Century Thought*, trans. David E. Green (New York: Holt, Rinehart and Winston, Inc., 1964) p. 6.

[34]Ibid. p. 3.

[35]Löwith remarks, moreover, that it would be mistaken to measure Hegel and Goethe by the achievements of their respective visions wrought at the hands of their students and disciples; this would be to underestimate the breadth and energy of their influence upon culture. Ibid. p.3.

[36] Sunlight p. xv.

[37]Kaufmann, *Hegel*, p. 134

[38]Ros. p. 99.

[39]Ibid. p. 381. Quoted in Kaufmann, *Hegel*, p. 239.

[40]Sunlight p. xxi. Despite his own suggestion Harris holds that Hegel first conceived himself to be a scholar and only later, through his acquaintance with Hölderlin, began to think along the lines of a *Volkserzieher.* See p. xix.

[41]Ibid. p. xxxi.

[42]Ibid. p. xxxii.

[43]Butler has made this point well with respect to Hegel's commitment to practical aims, even as he turns toward theoretical matters. Hegel, he maintains, engaged himself in practice precisely by transforming philosophy from a purely theoretical concern into a melding of theory and practice: "... there is a deepened understanding of philosophy as itself an expression of [practical] engagement." See, *Hegel: The Letters*, p. 65.

[44]Sunlight p. 6.

[45]Ibid.

[46]See Ros. pp. 7-21 and Sunlight pp. 7-44.

[47]For a fuller discussion of Hegel's characteristic idiosyncrasies as a student see Ros. p. 21ff.

[48]Ibid. p. 14.

[49]Ibid. p. 15.

[50]Sunlight p. 43.

[51]Ros. p. 178.

[52]See Kimmerle, *loc. cit.*

[53]See Findlay, *Hegel*, p. 31. Findlay puts it thus:

> "During this period [1803-1806] Hegel became less and less willing to hold that the crowning insights of philosophy could be arrived at by 'intuition', 'feeling' or suchlike immediate modes of experience: they must, he felt, emerge by a rational and necessary process, to which he now gave the time-honored name of 'Dialectic.'"

[54]Ros. p. 186. Quoted in translation by Cook, *Language*, p. 70.

[55]Ibid. p. 178.

[56]Hegel's comments specifically address the wholesale adoption of the Schellingian terminology by Schelling's students and followers.

[57]Ibid. 181.

[58]Ibid. p. 184. Harris and Knox give the likely date of the manuscript as 1805. See *System of Ethical Life*, p. 256, footnote. no. 3.

[59]Ros. p. 179.

[60]Night, p. 397f.

[61]Ibid. p. 398.

[62]See Ros. p. 15f, Sunlight p. 4ff, GB p. 14ff. Hegel's penchant for excerpting material will become an important issue as the discussion of his intellectual personality develops in subsequent sections of this investigation.

[63]Ros. p. 11f. According to Rosenkranz, Hegel's translations of Greek drama, stemming from his days in the Gymnasium at Stuttgart, the semimary at Tübingen, and Bern, remained a subject of great enthusiasm for him throughout his life. See also Harris's chronological appendix in Sunlight p. 47f and chronological index pp. 517-27.

[64]See his famous letter to Schelling of 1800 in *Hegel: The Letters*, p. 64.

[65]That there may be deeper problems with an account so dependent upon the practicality of Hegel's work is suggested by Rosenkranz's remark that: *Die Politik reizte ihn gewaltig, aber ein praktisches Eingreifen in dieselbe blieb ihm doch als That stets fern.* See. Ros. p. 21.

[66]The most obvious example of a subject Hegel taught in which he was not technically expert is the philosophy of nature. But this lack of training does not seem to compromise the value of his system of thought. That his though was applicable even in part to the sphere of nature is one of its most commendable aspects. Findlay, for example, has provided an eloquent defense for the importance of Hegel's philosophy of nature, both for understanding his system and on its own merit. See *Hegel*, p 267f.

[67]Ros. p. xxi.

[68]Ibid. p. xxxiii.

[69]The notion of a speculative Easter belongs not to Hegel but to Harris.

[70]Faith, p. 41. The Rosenkranz quotation comes from Ros., p. 141.

[71]Cerf and Harris, *System of Ethical Life and First Philosophy of Spirit*, p. 9. Harris argues in his introduction to the *First Philosophy of Spirit* (1803/04) that Hegel's insights into what became his mature system are developed in the new triadic conception of philosophy comprising the familiar encyclopaedic distinctions: I: Logic and Metaphysics, II: Philosophy of Nature, and III: Philosophy of Spirit. See p. 205, footnote no. 1, p. 7.

[72]*System of Ethical Life and First Philosophy of Spirit*, p. 7f.

[73]Harris implicitly admits as much in his identification of an emergent speculative philosophy in 1801. See ibid. p. 8f.

3

LEARNING: THE HERMENEUTICAL NEED OF PHILOSOPHY

In this chapter we will develop the theme of learning in Hegel's early philosophy. Before proceeding to this topic, however, allow me to briefly retrace the ground we have covered thus far. In Chapter One we saw how Hegel's concern with language led to the emergence of what we have come to know as his speculative discourse. We concluded that this unique form of expression provides his philosophy with its proper vehicle, and ultimately with its systematic articulation. In Chapter Two we investigated the biographical details of Hegel's nascent speculative discourse. We saw how the move to Jena marked the beginning of his career as a philosopher, and how the issue of language came into play with his speculative utterance of the death of God in 1802.

In the present chapter we will examine how the theme of language and the move to Jena fit in with the matter of learning. It is my hope here that we will gain an understanding of Hegel's commitment to explicating and promoting the perennial tradition of wisdom in Western culture. Specifically, we will learn that, according to Hegel's emergent conception of the history of thought and culture, his interest in language and his weighty decision to utter the death of God in Jena were not mere matters of his idiosyncrasy. Instead we will witness in his publications of this period his fervent conviction that the impetus of his thinking was in keeping with a higher necessity: the development of philosophy through speculative discourse fulfills the destiny of thought and culture as such.

Now, it is easy and even tempting in our present day to be suspicious of Hegel's grand designs. For even though he has in his favor two hundred years of tradition which present him as a pre-eminent thinker, still the general sense of scepticism, relativism, and more recently, cynicism which has become dominant in modern culture compels us to think that, no matter how great a mind he was, Hegel's thought is in the end a matter of personal opinion. But, as we will see, Hegel was not naive to such criticism. Though it is generally accepted that the 18th century was a time of great optimism, even of enlightenment, in European culture, he understood it to be infused with a debilitating form of relativism.[1] To be sure, the time was not then so characterized. And in terms of simple description, we could say that Hegel was just plain wrong. But, if we take into consideration his conception of culture, we will likely agree that Modernity was even then under the influence of a powerful, because latent, spirit of doubt and decline. Indeed, it was Hegel's considered judgment that the philosophy of the day, which was also the leading index of European culture at that time, was committed to the belief that there was no truth apart from personal opinion. So much was this the case, that the aim of philosophy, to seek wisdom, was undercut by an idle and weak-kneed scepticism. As witness to this, he pointed out how Fichte, one of the boldest thinkers in European culture at the time, was brought down on spurious charges of atheism. To one such as Hegel, trained in the history of the Western tradition, this debacle could not but call to mind the weakness of Athens manifest in its condemnation of Socrates or the cowardice of Rome displayed in Pilate's renunciation of the truth in the verdict against Jesus. In any case, Hegel was clear that the battle being fought against philosophy by philosophers themselves was the work of small minds. He set out to counter this tendency toward philosophical "apragmosyne", by turning it upon itself. And so he sounded a Faustian theme, expressing the weariness of the times, and the inertia of learning which was bequeathed to late Modernity by the Enlightenment. His assessment of philosophy and culture at the turn of the century is as follows:

> An age which has so many philosophical systems lying behind it in its
> past must apparently arrive at the same indifference which life acquires
> after it has tried all forms. (Diff. p. 85)

These words, which stand as the opening sentence of the introduction to his first philosophical publication echo the opening lines of Part One of Goethe's *Faust*:

> I've read, alas! through philosophy,
> Medicine and jurisprudence too,
> And, to my grief, theology
> With ardent labor studied through.
> And here I stand with all my lore,
> adept
> Poor fool, no wiser than before![2]

The difference between the young Hegel and the old Faust is that Hegel did not sell his soul to the devil for pleasure. Much rather, he committed himself to bringing learning to life.

In order for Hegel to accomplish his aim, it was necessary for him to come to terms with the then dominant philosophical tradition. The most imposing figure was Kant, for he had established the limits of knowledge in the theoretical, practical, and aesthetic spheres. His "critical philosophy" had spawned numerous attempts to refine the empirical thought of Locke and Hume. Hegel's position was that all such attempts undermined the true aim of philosophy. For, in manifold ways, they established a division between thinking and empirical reality. The latter was so priviledged in empiricism, that thought as such became problematic and sterile. To counter this tendency of late 18th century philosophy, Hegel had to demonstrate where things had gone wrong. He found it necessary to work within the terminology and systems of the broadly Kantian philosophy of the times, but to do so without succumbing to the obstacles inherent to that philosophy. His strategy was a bold one. He did not seek to avoid the pitfalls of parallogism and antinomy which dotted the landscape of the Kantian dialectic. Much rather he ventured to dive in head first, with the hope of penetrating the depths of the "abyss" of the Kantian system. He sensed intuitively, it seems, that if he succeeded, he would surface with a new philosophical perspective. That perspective was granted by his discovery of a speculative philosophy, a philosophy which was grounded not on the division between thinking and being (or in the Kantian terms, concept and intuition), but in their newfound identity.[3]

The development of Hegel's speculative thinking was presented in his first published essay, *Differenz des Fichte'schen und Schelling'schen Systems der Philosophie*.[4] In this important work Hegel introduces many of the issues and themes that dominate his later thought, perhaps the most enduring of which was his concern with philosophical method.[5] More than this, we will see that Hegel here outlines a genuinely hermeneutical approach to doing philosophy.[6] As others have noted, Hegel's concern with interpreting the history of philosophy in the *Differenz* essay is "prototypical" of his entire philosophical career.[7] And that career was distinguished by his unfailing concern with accounting for the whole. But this whole, for Hegel, is the expression of identity in difference, the core of his speculative philosophy. And so his (extensive) concern with the history of philosophy is his (intensive) concern with the whole of philosophy as the identity of its manifold parts. In this sense, philosophy is always *philosophia perennis*, for Hegel. But, as we will see, to pose the philosophical problem in this way, is to render it in a genuinely hermeneutical fashion. For, it is worth noting that Hegel did not attempt to deduce the whole of philosophical knowledge from a first principle, such as had been done with the Cartesian *cogito*. Nor did he proceed inductively, as had the empirical thinkers such as Locke. Instead he sought to interpret the history of philosophy as a series of parts, the whole of which was known, but known only intuitively. The whole which rendered the parts intelligible had to be arrived at by re-reading the history of philosophy as an unfolding of systems. In Hegel's way of putting it, this was to discover the "living spirit" which was articulated in the dead letter of philosophical texts.

This presentation of the problem of philosophy in the *Differenzschrift* resonates with Hegel's lifelong commitment to bring learning to life. As is apparent from his early youth, Hegel strove to become a lively interpreter of texts, or to put it more simply, to become an astute reader. We will see that even as a student in the gymnasium, Hegel was struggling to develop a vital understanding of the history of *les belles-lettres*. That learning is an essential part of life, and that life is the necessary form learning must take, are two propositions which might epitomize the formative strain of thought which at last comes to full expression in the *Differenzschrift*.

An analysis of this essay will provide a view of the young Hegel as a thinker who sought to repair the rift between learning and life he saw yawning before his critical gaze. Furthermore, because the *Differenzschrift* marked Hegel's debut in philosophical life[8], it provides the occasion to ask why he attempted to solve the general cultural problems of the day within the precincts of philosophy rather than in some other arena. The ranking of philosophy over religion and art which characterizes the mature Hegel finds its first justification here. Finally, the *Differenzschrift* anticipates the utterance of the death of God in the following year.[9] In the concluding passages of the essay he alludes to the death of God in saying: That which has died the death of dichotomy philosophy raises to life again through the absolute identity.[10] Thus the *Differenz* essay lays the groundwork for understanding this utterance at once as the critical evaluation of the accumulated cultural forms (art, religion, and, especially, philosophy) up to his time and as the evocation of a new and sufficient ideal of culture, namely, speculative discourse. The forum for this latter project (to be considered in subsequent chapters) was provided when Schelling, impressed by the *Differenzschrift*, invited Hegel to collaborate with him on the *Critical Journal of Philosophy*.[11]

A survey of the preface to the *Differenzschrift* will serve to identify the major issues of Hegel's general critique of culture and to introduce his speculative ideal. But before turning to these matters, we will examine a few brief selections from essays Hegel composed while in the gymnasium at Stuttgart. For in these the crucial elements of the *Differenzschrift* are prefigured.

Criticism and Speculation

The first essay to be considered presents Hegel's criticism of the accepted practice of translating passages from learned German works into Latin. Though Hegel acceded to the demands of his gymnasium teachers, and pursued this practice with industry, *"Über das Excipiren"*[12] shows clearly that he undertook his assignments with reservation and a characteristic reflection, which led him in all of his subsequent thinking. Hegel begins his essay by wondering why the practice of excerpting, *"die Niederschreibung eines Themas in einer andern Sprache, als in der das Thema abgefasst ist"*, is so heartily embraced by some and shunned by others. He notes that the proponents of this practice present it as a way of developing fluent Latin. It is the fluency of this Latin, however, which he challenges. For, he contends, when one considers the great differences between German constructions and those of other languages, it is apparent that the attempt to give German words and articles Latin clothes which are "far from Roman" obscures the *"Geist und Natur"* of the language itself.

According to his teachers, what counted as good Latin was the felicitous imitation of well-wrought words and phrases. What is left out, of course, are the various means of connecting words and the sequence of sentences. And this omission has the consequence of making language a mere exercise: *Von Sachen ist gar nicht die Rede.* Hegel sums up this point by noting that to take the greatest Latin stylists to be the best writers is to lead to "pompousness" and "bombast": *Das Natürliche und Aechte der Sprache wird ganz vernachlässigt.* Much rather one should prefer those authors who employ the less well-formed but richer constructions in language. For it is here that the strength of language is to be found.

Second, Hegel argues that the effortless selection of stylish phrases in excerpting a text leads to a lack of reflection: *Bei bekannten Worten braucht es freilich nicht viel Nachdenken.* This weakens one's grasp of language and weakens language's grasp on the world. It is better, he avers, to struggle to compose than to imitate freely. The strength of language, he concludes, can be discovered only through the repeated reading and interpretation of works written in foreign tongues.

Finally, he addresses the issue of criticism. Criticism, he contends, requires a mature grasp of language. The critic must drive at the living heart of a text, and avoid the pitfall of superficially adopting the author's own polished but dead phrases. Thus the philosophical study of language must accompany the practice of literary criticism.

The point in reviewing Hegel's essay is not to condemn the Latin language. Rather it is to see that even at the age of sixteen Hegel was compelled by the need to understand one's language by comparing it with another, preferably a classical one. He thus strove to bring language as such to bear on the problem of learning.

Aside from the resonances this piece has with the task formulated in Jena, to teach philosophy to speak German, it gives a brief view of the issue of criticism, as Hegel understood it at a very early age. His understanding of what constitutes genuine criticism, couched in the admission that such was not a proper subject for a youngster, is here clearly tied to the capacity of language to express the thing at hand (*die Sache selbst*). His impatience with the exercises at the Gymnasium is the same as that which spurs him to criticize the unnatural or technical language of philosophy in his Jena writings. Language is the living medium of thought and life itself. Thus dead language reflects the divorce of thinking and life, the demise of philosophy.

In another essay from the Gymnasium Hegel addresses the related topic of speculation. He begins "*Üeber die Religion der Griechen und Römer*"[13] with a consideration of the natural history of religion. The essay progresses through several simple stages until it arrives at the high point of Greek and Roman religion, namely, the emergence of a concept of divinity fashioned in regard to the fate of humankind: the divine has given each person the means to well-being and has so ordered things that true happiness can be found through wisdom and moral goodness. Here the analysis of religion becomes more original and sophisticated.

Hegel proposes that the sheer variety of speculative systems of thought developed in the ancient world to express the nature of divinity attests to the fact that the ancients struggled to find the proper form of truth. The observation he draws from this historical fact is that truth is often obscured through the habitual acceptance of given beliefs. When speculation ossifies into dogma, the truth is crushed. He counsels against allowing the spirit of speculation to be engulfed in the authority of entrenched opinions. Otherwise we will be powerless before our errors and half-truths. This note of hermeneutical suspicion, however, is balanced by a correlative charity in reading. The study of the historical forms of religion, he argues, awakens us from the slumber and lethargy which make us indifferent to truth, and hostile toward other cultures and peoples. For in the historical study of religion, we discover that many of our convictions are likely to be errors and that those of others may well be true. We come thus to judge other traditions more kindly and to understand them better.

This plea for toleration in religion, a commonplace of the Enlightenment tradition upon which the Stuttgart Gymnasium was based[14], has its source, for Hegel, in an appreciation for speculative thinking. The grounds for criticism, both of foreign and indigenous religious traditions, is the positive grasp of the divine enjoyed by those peoples who have achieved a philosophical culture. The characteristic errors of such peoples is not so much the inability to conceive the divine, but the failure to keep this conception alive through the influence of a bold speculative pursuit. When this pursuit is abandoned, humankind is fated to become entrapped in the stifling forms of received wisdom.

We might pause here to observe that, if Hegel's notions of the criticism of language, articulated in the essay on excerpting, and that of speculation upon the divine are correlated, it is easy to see how the young thinker found himself compelled to study seriously the Judeo-Christian tradition after he had left the Gymnasium.[15] For the sedimented creeds of this religious tradition, just as the polished phrases of the great Latin stylists, obscure the speculative efficacy of language. Thus a proper conception of the divine can be fostered and kept alive only by a careful criticism of the forms of language employed by this tradition. Those forms, collectively called *Vorstellungen* by the young Hegel, can be deemed to be errors or half-truths, or truth itself only by testing their speculative value. And speculative truth cannot be arrived at save through a genuinely philosophical consideration of the divine in its relation to the fate of humankind. Thus the task which emerges from fronting the fact of religious language is to grasp the history of philosophy as the chronicle of failed or genuine speculative insight. The fate of humankind, then, revolves around whether human culture dares to conceive of the divine in living language or chooses instead to smother the spirit of language in the stultifying forms of received wisdom. A bolder program of learning could hardly be imagined for a schoolboy.

Let me offer some general comments before passing on to the *Differenzschrift*. We have seen how Hegel's habits of reading helped him to arrive at a certain interpretation of Western culture. He was both an insatiable and a strong reader, and these qualities enabled him to remain speculative, to see beyond the limitations of any given text, even as he criticized its forms. He developed a practice of reading which would serve him his entire life. The texts of Western culture did not represent to him the simple, encyclopaedic unfolding of knowledge, as was the working assumption of the Enlightenment. Rather, they presented cyclic and mounting tensions which were seen to erupt from time to time in the form of cultural crises. The rise and fall of Greek and then Roman culture; the emergence and schism of the Christian church; the birth of modernity and its impending demise at the end of the 18th century; these were the most obvious transformations. But beneath and between them were myriad permutations of the same basic tensions of culture. Once these crises were brought to speech, articulated, cut at the joints, the entire Western tradition could be read in the light of a speculative paradigm. As we will see, the utterance of the death of God in 1802 would both reveal and anticipate a solution to the pre-eminent crisis of modern times. But before this utterance could be formed, it was necessary to take stock of the age. This Hegel set out to do in the *Differenzschrift*. For his task he employed tools which were by then his familiar friends, namely, criticism and speculation.

Difference

By the time Hegel undertook to criticize and speculate upon the culture of modernity in the *Differenzschrift*, he had become an adept in philosophy. And this with good reason, for his sojourns in the realms of art and religion had taught him that the modern period, in contrast to other epochs in Western culture, was uniquely philosophical in kind. Thus he pursued the question of the times in relation to the philosophical systems of the age.[16] In the preface and introduction to the essay he lays out the basic problems to be dealt with. But, to the uninitiated, these are extremely difficult indeed. At the risk of being pedantic, let me offer an explanation of the crucial distinction between reflection and speculation. Then I will list some of the more important terms which orbit around that distinction.

As mentioned above, Hegel delves into the philosophy of his day with a view to overturning it. What we have generally refered to as Kantianism or the critical philosophy, Hegel most often calls the philosophy of reflection (*Reflexionsphilosophie*). He employs the basic terminology of this philosophy, but he does so from the perspective of speculative philosophy. What this means in practical terms is that things get unbelievably confused. What meant one thing for Kant, means two things for Hegel. But there is a way through this thicket of terminology, though it cannot leave the reader unscathed. The key is to see that, for Hegel, the philosophy of reflection is made up of inherent oppositions, whereas speculative philosophy is rooted in identity (though not without inherent differences!) To clear a bit of a path, permit me to comment, as others often have, on the difference between reflection (*Reflexion*) and speculation (*Spekulation*).[17]

The distinction between these two technical terms is crucial, yet difficult to grasp. The difficulty arises because, in their root senses, the words mean basically the same thing. They both have to do with the relation between an original something and its image. This is obvious in the case of reflection, but less so with respect to speculation, until one recognizes that the Latin root of the word is the name for a mirror (*speculum*). The question is, How is the relation between original and image different in reflection and speculation? Let us begin with reflection. When something is reflected in a mirror, its image is presented as a copy of an object, a thing. Thus to speak of reflection is to speak of the formal difference between the original and the image, even if that difference is in the form of correspondence, i.e., the image is the reflection *of* the original. Generally there is here a priority for the original over the image, since the image is the mere appearance of the thing itself. Speculation, on the other hand, is the insight of looking into the mirror, or speculum. This is apparent in the Latin verbal root, *speculor*, which means to look. Here it is neither the image nor the original which is primary. Hence the difference (correspondence) between the two is not primary either. Instead the interplay (which, as we will see, is infinite in this case) between the mirror as a reflecting surface and the eye as a reflecting surface is primary. When one looks in the mirror, one can see this —the act of seeing itself— which is also a knowing (i.e., recognition). But one can also fail to see this. One might see only one's reflection. And so we find ourselves back in reflection.

The ways in which speculation fails, that is to say, the ways in which it turns into reflection are revealing, for they show us the real difference between reflection and speculation. When one looks in the mirror and sees one's reflection, perhaps one is struck by the difference manifest even within this correspondence of original and image. One might think, This does not look like me. In extreme cases, there is a confusion between the mental image (which here serves as the original) and the mirror image. The difference between the mental image and the mirror image might, for example, lead to narcissism, as in the myth of Narcissus. The problem here, of course, is that the beautiful lad has such a defective mental image of himself, that he falls in love with his mirror image, thinking it is another. Of a more mundane sort, is the experience we have all had of looking in the mirror and failing to recognize ourselves therein. This could be in a figurative way, as when we say that we looked in the mirror and did not recognize the person we had become. But also in a quite literal sense, we might look in the mirror (generally this happens in the morning) and express shock at what we see. Or perhaps the difference between our mental image of ourselves and our mirror image might be a matter of humor, as when we make faces in the mirror. Finally, this difference might be a matter of simple indifference or detachment. But in each case the structure of difference is primary, and so we know we are dealing with reflection. Thus, at best, looking at the image of oneself in the mirror presents a special case of looking at images, or mere appearances. But it is never an instance of speculation. Not until it becomes a case of looking at looking.

Notice too how reflection can go wrong in another interesting way. It could happen that reflection grows tired of the subjectivity of looking at one's own image, and the compromised objectivity of looking at the image of other things, and holds up a mirror to the mirror. The spectacle of reflection here is intriguing. The mirrors play the empty images of each other back and forth *ad infinitum*. But what have we here? A house of mirrors. An image of nihilism.[18]

The Scylla and Charybdis of reflection, namely, narcissism and nihilism, can only be avoided by keeping the speculum of the eye itself in the picture. Looking at oneself and playing with mirrors can be avoided when one intuits and sees the infinite play of the eye in the mirror. For here one sees and knows the I, and not merely as a thing which sees, but also as a knowing. An interesting consequence of this is that the image of oneself must be given up in seeing insight itself, for of necessity, to see the speculum of the eye, the image of oneself must be out of focus. To demonstrate this, assume an ordinary pose in front of a mirror. You have a good view of yourself. But you are much too far away to see anything else. Now approach the mirror. Get as close as you can, so that you can see the reflection of one of your eyes up close. Notice the tiny image of yourself which is reflected on your pupil. Now think: What you are seeing is an image of yourself reflected in your eye, which is in turn reflected back to your eye from the surface of the mirror in front of you. And nothing else. You cannot properly see your own image in the mirror at this point. In a sense, you cannot even think that image either. For your intuition has already told you that, within the speculum of the eye belonging to that tiny image of yourself, there must be a much smaller, even an invisible, image of yourself. And so on, *ad infinitum, ad infinitesimum.* Notice also that in this interplay of mirror and eye, one cannot become infatuated with the interplay of empty images, as in the nihilistic act of holding a mirror up to a mirror. This is because the play of images is never empty (it always includes an image of yourself looking) and because the play of images recede in scale so dramatically that you cannot see past the image (in your eye's speculum) of yourself looking. That is just the way it is. But this is fortunate, it seems, because it is a sure way around narcissism. The flat surface of water (our original mirror) reflects the image of the eye's speculum in such a way that we cannot see the miniscule image of the self in it. It is just too small. And we could hardly fall in love with this Lilliputian self anyway!

Now, back to Hegel. To understand the distinction between reflection and speculation we need only recognize that reflection is forever caught within the difference (Hegel says, opposition) between the original and the image, or, in the case of Kant, the thing-in-itself and its appearance. But speculation recognizes that the image and the original are identical in the act of looking. In more properly Hegelian terms, we would say that reflection is the mere appearance of speculation.[19] However, there are in philosophy a thousand ways of missing this basic truth. For this reason, speculation may succumb to reflection.

The oppositions which constitute the philosophy of reflection are legion. A few of the more important ones mentioned by Hegel are as follows:

Subject/Object
Reason/Understanding
Noumena/Phenomena
Thought/Being
Freedom/Nature
Mind/Body
Spirit/Matter
God/World/Man
Universality/Particularity
Infinite/Finite
Eternity/Present
Intelligible/Sensible
Intuition/Concept
Ideal/Real

To this list Hegel adds a host of other distinctions which are meant to distinguish speculative philosophy from the philosophy of reflection. A few of these are as follows:

Speculation/Reflection
Absolute Identity/ Infinite Opposition
Idea/Being
True Infinity/Chain of Finite Acts and Objects
Absolute Self-Intuition/Ego
Inner Necessity/Need of the Times
Reason/Nature
Subjective Subject-Object/Objective Subject-Object
Totality/Completeness of Information
Individuality/Life
Philosophy/Information, Opinion, Erudition, Appearance
Philosophy/Philosophical Systems
Living Spirit/Dead Opinion
Absolute/Reason
Philosophical Speculation/Reason, Living Originality of Spirit/Dichotomy
Being/Non-Being
Absolute Itself/Dichotomy
Absolute/Reflection
Conscious/Non-Conscious
Determinate/Indeterminate

Part/Whole
Speculation/Common Sense
Feeling/Faith
Matter/Life
A/A
Reflection/Intuition
History of the One/Tales of Opinions

This list differs from the previous one not only with respect to its content, but also and more importantly in that the relation between the terms is not often one of opposition. This is most apparent when one considers a list of terms (drawn from both of the lists above) which are manifestly speculative in kind. For this list shows that Hegel often is at pains to underscore the identity within the difference of certain terms. A few of his "speculative" terms are as follows:

Individuality: universality/particularity
Becoming: being/non-being
Appearance: Absolute itself/dichotomy
Life: finite/infinite
Contradiction: Absolute/reflection
Knowledge: intelligible/sensuous
Standing: whole/part
Feeling: unlimited/limited
Faith: unlimited/limited
Transcedental Knowledge: concept/being
Time: eternity/present
History of Philosophy: history of the One/tales of opinions

The usefulness of this list is that it shows in a cursory way how Hegel sought to think the coincidence of opposites. To this end he employed many figures of speech, some of which are quite remarkable. Rather than providing yet another list, however, I will summarize. The figures of speech meant to articulate these *coincidentia oppositorum* dispell the common assumption that Hegelian opposites are melded together in 'syntheses'. Rather they are held together in dynamic combinations of free radicals. The force of the *relata* necessitates that the binding and unbinding of combinations involves a good deal of fireworks. Accordingly, Hegel's figures of speech are mostly drawn from images of death and destruction (e.g., cobwebs, mummies, fossils, deafness, abyss, night, shipwreck, death etc.) A few are drawn from life (e.g., voice, living spirit, harmony, light, etc.). What is revealing about Hegel's use of these figures of speech is that they conspire to tell a dramatic tale of the "fate of philosophy" (another of his figures of speech!) But before turning to that tale, allow me to provide a brief sketch of the critical project of the *Differnzschrift* as Hegel presented it.

The superficial[20] occasion for the essay is the fact that many failed, in Hegel's judgment, to distinguish between the philosophical systems of Fichte and Schelling. Most especially, Reinhold had failed to differentiate the two systems of idealism in his endorsement of a philosophical revolution which was to bring philosophy back to logic.[21] The confusion of these two systems was apparently the justification for such a revolution. By properly distinguishing Fichte's and Schelling's respective contributions, Hegel hoped to show the mistake of the turn back to logic, which precluded the true appropriation of the Kantian critical philosophy and the proper development of philosophy as such.

Hegel's strategy is to demonstrate the presence of a truly speculative principle underlying the surface of Kant's philosophy:

> The Kantian philosophy needed to have its spirit distinguished from its letter, and to have its purely speculative principle lifted out of the remainder that belonged to, or could be used for, the arguments of reflection. (Diff., p. 79)

Fichte, Hegel maintains, is responsible for extracting this principle from the Kantian deduction of the categories, and presenting it in the form of an authentic idealism. The principle in question is the identity of subject and object presented in the deduction of the forms of understanding.[22] This identity is, according to Hegel, reason itself, and it was turned by Kant into the object of philosophical reflection. But, by rendering such identity as an **object**, Kant had driven a wedge deep within the heart of reason, thus destroying the identity. Reason then came to be replaced by the realm of appearance. The effect is that reason (the identity of subject and object) is subjugated to the understanding.[23]

The subjugation of reason to understanding has two steps in the Kantian philosophy, according to Hegel. First the identity of subject and object is limited to the acts of thinking represented by the categories of the understanding. Second, aside from what is objectively determined by the concepts of the understanding in the first step, there remains a limitless empirical region of the sensible and perception. This region Hegel calls an absolute *aposteriority*, which is determined only by the subjective maxims of reflective judgment.[24] Because the maxims of judgment are merely subjective, Hegel argues, the identity of subject and object becomes a non-identity, raised to an absolute principle. This was to be expected from a philosophy which conceived of reason as practical, for practical reason is not the identity of subject and object, but rather the mere unity of the understanding opposed to the finitude of the sensible.[25]

The principle of Fichte's system is the identity of subject and object. The original Kantian insight into this identity is expressed in Fichte's formula: *Ich = Ich*.[26] This, according to Hegel, is the bold expression of the genuine principle of speculation. But, Hegel notes, Fichte abandons this principle as soon as he begins to develop his system from out of it.[27] The result, according to Hegel, is that the I does not constitute itself in absolute self-intuition. Thus the formula I=I is transformed into the principle, I *ought* to be equal to I. The disparity signified by this subjunctive[28] involves a progression *ad infinitum* in which the I is never delivered from temporal succession. Reason, thus debased, is expressed in the shapes of the understanding that the absolute must take upon itself. Knowledge, therefore, is construed as the science of the finite shapes of the absolute.[29]

Hegel points out that Fichte's philosophy has two sides. On one hand, it posits the identity of subject and object, and so renders philosophy possible. On the other hand, this identity (Reason) is grasped by Fichte in the form of pure consciousness (the self). Thus the finite principle of the self is raised to an absolute level. The task Hegel takes upon himself is to demonstrate that the necessity of the thing itself (*die Sache selbst*) determines that reason cannot finally be identified with pure consciousness.

Hegel proffers Schelling's philosophy of nature as the basis for drawing such a distinction between reason and the self. For, by discovering the identity of subject and object in nature as well as in the self, Schelling avoids the Fichtean pitfall of subjectivism. Schelling, Hegel holds, finds the identity of subject and object, self and nature, in something higher than both.[30] That "something higher" is the telos of Hegel's essay.

The Fate of Reason

But the pursuit of this telos involves, for Hegel, an account of why philosophy has fallen into the trap of identifying reason with the finite form of the self. The explanation is to be found in the conception of philosophy that Hegel presents here. The fate of philosophy is that thinking is a living form, subject to the vicissitudes of history, reflected in human freedom. This fate was, according to Hegel, dramatically manifest in his time: the dissolution of life into systematic paralysis is the necessary outcome of the history of thought. All philosophy has become opinion; in some sense it is always passé.[31] That philosophical systems are obsolete as soon as they come off the press is a result not of the limitations of human cognition, so much as of the inherently historical nature of philosophy itself. It is the fate of the one eternal philosophy that it has to enter into time, in a particular place, and in the form of a particular system:

> As every living form belongs at the same time to the realm of appearance, so too does philosophy. (Ibid., p. 85)

This dictates that philosophy must respond to something (other than itself) already in place. If it responds by reflecting upon that something as the object of thought, it must suffer an unhappy fate:

> As appearance, philosophy surrenders to the power capable of transforming it into dead opinion and into something that belonged to the past from the very beginning. (Ibid., p. 85f.)

But, as we will soon see, if that something other is taken to be the appearance of philosophy in time, then philosophy and its other are united in the form of speculation.[32]

  The transience of philosophical systems is to be contrasted to the living spirit of philosophy. For, accoring to Hegel, there is a spirit which dwells within the house of philosophy. And this spirit will unveil itself to a kindred spirit. But to opinionizers it remains concealed.[33] And, though the spirit of philosophy itself suffers no harm from the opinions of philosophers, the philosopher is nothing without this spirit.

  There is, however, the possibility that philosophers —the "big brains", as Hegel calls them— can take the proper approach to thinking:

> But if the Absolute, like Reason which is its appearance, is eternally one and the same—as indeed it is—then every Reason that is directed toward itself and comes to recognize itself, produces a true philosophy and solves for itself the problem which, like its solution, is at all times the same. (Ibid., p. 87)

With reason as the true subject of philosophy, or rather when philosophical systems are constructed out of reason itself, the Absolute[34] finds its adequate expression. Therein the shackles of historical vicissitudes are thrown off, and the philosopher is delivered from the realm of mere opinion. At the same time spirit is made free for philosophy; philosophy discovers its inner essence. For, in the true appearance of the Absolute, reason is eternal[35]; the philosopher and spirit are one. Thus the history of philosophy reveals that, when it comes to the essence of philosophy, there are neither predecessors nor successors.[36]

Hegel's distinction between reason and opinion reflects the two sides of philosophy. On one hand, knowledge is bound by history, opinion, and personal idiosyncrasies. On the other hand, freed from its outward forms, it is one and eternally the same. The systems of philosophy, Hegel holds, belong to the transient forms of thinking, the realm of opinion, while the essence of philosophy pertains to the inner truth of the Absolute. And the way which leads from the history of thinking to its eternal form, from opinion to philosophy, is littered with the wrecked ships of would-be philosophers, run aground by helmsmen who have become distracted by opinion.

Yet, despite the warning of so great a system builder as Kant,[37] Hegel counsels against staying put on the island of opinions, imploring that we must venture forth upon the sea of thought, in search of a more suitable landfall:

> —for though we see that the shores of those philosophical Islands of the Blest that we yearn for are only littered with the hulks of wrecked ships, and there is no vessel safe at anchor in their bays, yet we must not let go of the teleological perspective. (Ibid., p. 87)

The voyage to the paradisical island of truth is a dangerous one indeed, according to Hegel, and the passage will not be without casualties. Still, one must sacrifice oneself to the stormy seas.[38] One must respond to the initiative of philosophy to enter into time by letting go of one's historically bound opinions.

The tide which bears Hegel's philosophical vessel out to sea is speculation. Speculation, Hegel proffers, is the activity of singular, universal reason.[39] It is the force of thinking itself which liberates the philosopher from the bounds of common consciousness.[40] Once one is thus freed for thinking, a philosophical system can be articulated which will bring speculation into its own. For in the shapes assumed by speculative thinking, philosophy can find its completion.[41] But, it is important to note here that the "vessel" Hegel employs is not itself a system of philosophy. Much rather it is an approach for critically and speculatively interpreting this history of system building. The model he utilizes for reading philosophy is as follows:

> Every philosophy is complete in itself, and like an authentic work of art, carries the totality within itself. Just as the works of Apelles or Sophocles would not have appeared to Raphael and Shakespeare—had they known of them—as mere preparatory studies, but as a kindred force of the spirit, so Reason cannot regard its former shapes as merely useful preludes to itself. Virgil, to be sure, regarded Homer to be such a prelude to himself and his refined era, and for this reason Virgil's work remains a mere postlude. (Ibid., p. 89)

The Need of Philosophy

This model for reading is rooted in Hegel's important notion of the need of philosophy (*Bedürfnis der Philosophie.*) Philosophy, even as a great work of art, stands in need of renaissance. But, such a renaissance cannot take place unless, first, there is a need for philosophy in the culture of the times, and second, there is a need within philosophy itself which will be met through its rebirth. These two aspects of the need of philosophy are rooted in a grammatical ambiguity of some consequence to Hegel's thinking.[42]

The genetive in the phrase, *das Bedürfnis der Philosophie*, functions both objectively and subjectively. In the former sense, the need of philosophy denotes a general cultural need for a proper philosophical system. In the latter sense, the phrase denotes a need within philosophy itself, a lack or failing inherent to philosophy. The need for philosophy is the particular form for the general condition Hegel refered to as the "need of the times" (*Zeitbedürfnis.*) The need within philosophy is the general name for the particular condition Hegel called the "inner necessity of the thing itself" (*innere Notwendigkeit der Sache selbst.*)[43]

Both of these aspects of the need of philosophy are rooted in what Hegel calls dichotomy (*Entzweiung.*) Dichotomy, the sundering of harmonies, is a "... factor in life."[44] It works itself out in many ways in culture:

> As culture grows and spreads, and the development of those outward expressions of life into which dichotomy can entwine itself becomes more manifold, the power of dichotomy becomes greater, its regional sanctity is more firmly established and the strivings of life to give birth once more to its harmony become more meaningless, more alien to the cultural whole. (Ibid., p. 92)

One of the many cultural forms that dichtomy assumes is philosophy. Thus the need within philosophy is a special form which has emerged in culture.

> Antitheses such as spirit and matter, soul and body, faith and intellect, freedom and necessity, etc. used to be important; and in more limited spheres they appeared in a variety of other guises. The whole weight of human interests hung upon them. With the progress of culture they have passed over into such forms as the antithesis of Reason and sensibility, intelligence and nature and, with respect to the universal concept, of absolute subjectivity and objectivity. (Ibid., p. 90)

We can see, then, that the need within philosophy reflects the dichotomies produced by culture. What sense does it make to say that there is a need within culture for philosophy? Hegel's answer is as follows:

> If we look more closely at the particular form worn by a philosophy we see that it arises, on the one hand, from the living originality of the spirit whose work and spontaneity have reestablished and shaped the harmony that has been rent; and on the other hand, from the particular form of the dichotomy from which the system emerges. (Ibid., p. 89)

In other words, philosophy arises as a solution to the problem of dichotomy in culture, and yet it has dichotomy within itself. But there is a transition here. Hegel avers that the former sort of dichotomy is contingent, while the latter is necessary. This distinction helps Hegel to discover a way of meeting both species of need.

Hegel rehearses what he takes to be the development of the contingent forms of the dichotomy upon which culture rests. Then he shows how the latest of these forms is in fact a necessary dichotomy. He begins by breaking the development down into its component elements, the first of which is art:

> The entire system of relations constituting life has become detached from art, and thus the concept of art's all-embracing coherence has been lost, and transformed into the concept either of superstition or of entertainment.[45]

The next element, religion, takes up what remains of art:

> The highest aesthetic perfection, as it evolves in a determinate religion in which man lifts himself above all dichotomy and sees both the freedom of the subject and the necessity of the object vanish in the kingdom of grace, could only be energized up to a certain stage of culture, and within general or mob barbarism. As it progressed, civilization has split away from it [i.e., this aesthetic religious perfection], and juxtaposed it to itself or vice versa.[46]

The next, and penultimate, stage of this progression marks the emergence of philosophy as a cultural form, but one which is still contingent:

> When, where and in what forms such self-productions of Reason occur as philosophies is contingent. ... In the form of fixed reflection, as a world of thinking and thought essence in antitheses to a world of actuality, this dichotomy falls into the Northwest.[47]

Once dichotomy has assumed the form of philosophy, it is not long before its necessity becomes apparent.[48]

Let us take a moment to summarize and ponder Hegel's notion of the need of philosophy. We have come to the point where we can understand how the philosophical distinction between subject and object has developed into a dichotomy which is the manifestation of another, more general rift between learning and the living originality of spirit. But we might wonder how this distinction can in any way serve to meet the needs of culture. Indeed, on the face of it, Hegel's suggestion seems absurd. For consider the situation. Hegel is describing the 18th century (or modernity in general) as a time which has a peculiar species of need, namely, it lacks a solution to the patently philosophical problem of the subject/ object dichotomy. But it seems that when philosophy lends a hand, things only get worse. When the philosophy of reflection arises in response to the need of the times, it serves to intensify that need rather than satisfy it. When the masses cried out in hunger for bread, Marie Antoinette said supposedly, Let them eat cake. When they wanted a little milk to go with it, Kant said, I'll milk the he-goat if you'll hold the sieve.

It is not to stretch matters too much to say that the philosophers of the day had indeed turned their backs on the needs of the culture. When the people yearned for truth, they were given the considered opinion that there was none. But Hegel would have none of this. He came up against the absolute necessity of dichotomy in philosophy, and set out to transform dichotomy into a philosophical form which would indeed meet the need of the times. He would not allow the failure of philosophy to become the death of thinking.

His strategy was to learn from the great failures of culture. For he knew that the need of philosophy had arisen because, first, the artistic and, then, the religious expressions of culture had become inadequate for life. When the Classical artistic ideal was supplanted by Christianity, it became out-moded and defunct, despite many attempts at renaissance and rebirth. Likewise, when catholic religion was overturned in the Protestant Reformation, religion itself became moribund as a cultural form. Thus arose the need for philosophy, a new form of cultural expression, dedicated to the same end as the other forms, namely, expressing the unity of God and the world.

But Hegel knew well this could have been otherwise. Allow me to elaborate. Had history not taken the turns its did, had Constantine not adopted Christianity, had Luther not nailed his theses upon the cathedral door, philosophy as such simply would not have arisen in modern Europe. For philosophy, Hegel argued, arises only when it is needed. However, that philosophy should display its own species of need when it did arise was no mere matter of contingency. If and when philosophy appears, it must of necessity appear as dichotomy. Could Descartes have asked another, a non-philosophical, question? Indubitably. Shakespeare and Cervantes did. Montaigne and Erasmus did as well. But could philosophy assume any other form in Descartes besides the division of mind and body, subject and object? Manifestly not. By virtue of asking about thinking, Descartes led us into the uniquely modern labyrinth of absolute dichotomy. It fell to Hegel to attempt a way out.

His method was to tackle dichotomy head on. He sought to demonstrate that philosophy had only managed to address the world of appearance and not the identity of appearance and the Absolute. If he succeeded in establishing this basic insight, it would become clear that dichotomy reigned supreme in philosophy only because no one had yet constructed a philosophical system based on the identity of opposites.

When philosophy fails to see the whole of appearance for what it is, it becomes a detriment to itself and to culture. This failure occurs when philosophy limits itself to the sphere of appearance through the employment of the understanding, the supreme faculty of the philosophy of reflection. Philosophy focusses upon the ability of the understanding to set its own limits, and so expands the realm of appearance *ad infinitum.* Philosophy thus erects a Tower of Babel of sorts: in attempting to construct a vantage point in the understanding from which it hopes to view the whole of appearance, it divorces itself from the one thing that can provide the realm of appearance its true totality, namely, the Absolute.[49]

The need of philosophy is met through discovering the totality of thinking from out of the manifold of appearance, not by equating the whole with the sphere of appearance:

> Reason reaches the Absolute only in stepping out of this manifold of
> parts. (Ibid., p. 89f.)

But the attempt to break through the whole of appearance into the true totality of the Absolute is hindered, in Hegel's estimation, by philosophical vanity and its insistence upon the power of understanding. Yet, even as philosophy comes more and more to rely upon understanding, culture becomes more restless in its search for the Absolute.[50] This restlessness is calmed only through the pursuit of reason, for reason, as the vehicle of speculative philosophy, has the power to suspend the ceaseless toil of the understanding.   Hegel thus posits reason as the form in which the need of philosophy is met. The grasp of the Absolute frees philosophy for its true form, speculation, and liberates life from the bonds of mere appearance. Thus culture, as the divorce of life and learning, is transformed into the pursuit of the Absolute.

The need of philosophy is to be met through a proper grasp of the relation between reason and understanding, speculative philosophy and the philosophy of reflection. Understanding, Hegel maintains, is an imitation of reason. Whereas reason posits the identity of subject and object, understanding merely seems to posit such identities. In the case of the relation of the finite and the infinite, for example, understanding isolates the aspect of negation in reason[51], and so conceives of the infinite as the negation of the finite. In so doing, reflective thinking lowers reason to the level of understanding and its oppositions. To grasp the procession of these oppositions of understanding is the proper aim of reason. For only through reason can the identity presupposed by such oppositions be exposed. In the infinite activity of reason the oppositions are united in the original totality which conditions them.[52]

The way in which Hegel attempts to account for the need within philosophy is to say that it is the presupposition of the understanding, or the philosophy of reflection. He first depicts this in the figurative language of a battle between reason and the understanding. This description ties in with the discussion of the fate of philosophy above. This fate provides the final justification for Hegel's claim that the need within philosophy is a matter of necessity:

> In the struggle of the intellect [i.e. understanding] with Reason the intellect has strength only to the degree that Reason forsakes itself. Its success in the struggle therefore depends upon Reason itself, and upon the authenticity of the need for the reconstitution of totality, the need from which Reason emerges. (Ibid., p. 93)

Thus reason engages the understanding only because of the need which arises from the necessity of the opposition between subject and object. The understanding achieves a relative victory over reason only because reason has sundered itself. The origin of the opposition between subject and object is, therefore, not understanding, but the division within the Absolute itself. And only when reason allows that opposition to become absolute in the form of the understanding, does the necessity of the opposition become apparent to understanding. Once this much is manifest, the contingent need of the philosophy of the understanding, namely, the philosophy of reflection, to attain to totality is seen to rest upon the necessary need of philosophy, or reason, to return[53] to the totality of the Absolute. Hegel expresses it as follows:

> The need of philosophy can be called the *presupposition* of philosophy if philosophy, which begins with itself, has to be furnished with some sort of vestibule .... What is called the presupposition of philosophy is nothing else but the need that has come to utterance.

The point here is that the need of philosophy to attain to totality, as posited by the philosophy of reflection, is contingent, but, when considered as a presupposition, the need of philosophy to return to the totality of the Absolute is seen in its necessity.

But, when the need of philosophy is posited by the philosophy of reflection, its presupposition takes on the twofold form of reflection. On one hand, the need of philosophy is the Absolute itself, that for which philosophy seeks. On the other hand, it is that which philosophy seeks to overcome, namely, the dichotomies of being and not-being, concept and being, finitude and infinity.[54] Hegel portrays the relationship between these presuppositions of reflection in the form of a metaphor:

> The Absolute is the night, and the light is younger than it; and the distinction between them, like the emergence of the light out of the night, is an absolute difference—the nothing is the first out of which all being, all the manifoldness of the finite has emerged.

However, Hegel presses, the task of philosophy is to unite these presuppositions:

> But the task of philosophy consists in uniting these presuppositions: to posit being in non-being, as becoming; to posit dichotomy in the Absolute, as its appearance; to posit the finite in the infinite, as life. (Ibid., p. 93f.)

Thus the distinction between the Absolute and reflective consciousness is suspended in the metaphor: the night of the Absolute grows into the daylight of consciousness. But this is to pose the matter from the perspective of the contingent, and so the difference between them is absolute.

If the Absolute and consciousness are not merely to be seen contingently, as in the metaphor of day breaking forth from night, how is their union to be understood? The passage in question is obviously not too clear. However, a suggestion seems to come from the final pair, the finite and the infinite. If we skip over the previous two pairs, Hegel's statement would read: The task of philosophy consists in uniting these two presuppositions; to posit the finite in the infinite—as life. The grammar of the sentence would dictate that the finite is to be posed as the infinite.[55] Accordingly life would be conceived as the infinity of the finite. And this is in keeping with Hegel's general notion that the finite forms of understanding expressed in culture, namely, learning, must be seen to pass over into life. The task of philosophy, then, is to bring learning to life, and not merely in the sense of making learning practical, but more significantly in the sense of enlivening learning.[56] It is precisely this latter sense which informs Hegel's analysis of the philosophy of reflection in the next section of his essay.

Reflection

In this section Hegel portrays reflection as the instrument employed in the philosophical task outlined above. Learning is enlivened through the demise of the understanding; reason is set free when, finally, understanding loosens its grip upon reflection.[57] The need of philosophy (in both senses of the term) is that the Absolute should be constituted for consciousness. But the production of the Absolute in *Reflexion*, i.e., becoming, and the Absolute as the product of *Reflexion*, i.e., appearance, are both mere limits, according to Hegel. Thus the need of philosophy expressed as presupposition is a contradiction.[58] The contradiction lies in positing the Absolute as the twofold limit of *Reflexion*, as that which conditions and is conditioned by consciousness.[59] But, Hegel continues, the mediation of this contradiction is just the philosophical aspect of *Reflexion* which he seeks here to expose. Hegel elaborates upon the justification of this fundamental task:

> Reflection in isolation is the positing of opposites, and this would be a suspension of the Absolute ....

Insofar as the limited has standing, Hegel notes, reason is presented as the power of the negative Absolute. As such it is an absolute negating of the limited. At the same time, however, it is still the power of positing. In this capacity, reason poses the opposition of the objective and the subjective in the totality of the Absolute.

In the capacity of the negative Absolute, reason seduces the understanding (the faculty of limitations) into producing an objective totality.[60] What here appears to be the effect of *Reflexion* bound by understanding, Hegel points out, is in truth the secret efficacy of reason to attain a necessary totality:

> Reason makes the intellect boundless, and in this infinite wealth the intellect and its objective world meet their downfall. For every being that the intellect produces is something determinate, and the determinate has an indeterminate before and after it. The manifoldness of being lies between two nights, without support. It rests on nothing ... (Ibid., p. 95)

Reason thus threatens to engulf the objective world of the understanding in the abyss of the unconditioned. The finitude of the understanding floats upon a dark sea of infinity. Poised precariously, the understanding makes its final futile gesture; it grants the distinction between the finite and the infinite, and attempts to hold itself fast to the former. But here the contest is decided:

If the intellect fixes these opposites, the finite and the infinite, so that both are supposed to subsist together as opposed to each other, then it destroys itself. For the opposition of finite and infinite means that to posit the one is to cancel the other. Recognizing the mutually exclusive opposition of the finite and the infinite, as posed by a desperate understanding, reason is resolved to its task. The pitch of the battle is at hand; understanding is helpless before its foe. The throat is bared, and reason hesitates not in dealing the fatal blow. Reason destroys the understanding.

We might feel here that Hegel has expressed a rather dreadful thought. But this, only if we fail to see the necessity of the affair. Reason, having once risked itself upon the "field of battle", having entered into *Reflexion*, is now powerless to alter the rules of the contest. The battle is unto the death; to relent would be only to perpetuate the conflict. But understanding has justly fallen to reason in accord with the immutable law of *Reflexion*:

> So far as reflection makes itself it own object, its supreme law, given to it by Reason and moving it to become Reason, is to nullify itself. (Ibid., p. 96)[61]

According to Hegel, once understanding has sundered itself, *Reflexion* is transformed into speculation, and philosophy achieves its proper standpoint. The problems of *Reflexion* which stem from the understanding have dissolved. Now reason is free to think.[62] This is the way in which the need of philosophy is met. Speculation grasps the unity of opposites as the whole of knowledge. And this is the systematic basis for thought. Hegel describes this basis in the language of the part and the whole:

> Within this organization, every part is at the same time the whole; for its standing is its connection with the Absolute. As a part that has other parts outside of it, it is something limited, and is only through the others. Isolated in its limitation the part is defective; meaning and significance it has solely through its coherence with the whole. (Ibid., p. 98)

Hermeneutics

Hegel's conception of the relation of the part and whole in knowledge is the foundation of his speculative philosophy. Accordingly, it warrants further attention. What I hope to establish in this context is that the need of philosophy is hermeneutical in kind, that philosophy can only be understood as the text-bound relation between the part and the whole.

This suggestion might strike the reader as implausible. And, on its surface, it is indeed odd to speak of Hegel in relation to the science of intepretation, for he nowhere associates himself with the modern revival of hermeneutics in the late eighteenth-century Germany. Furthermore, the matter of interpretation was in that period limited to the sphere of biblical, literary, and legal texts, and did not come into play in philosophical writings. But, as we will see, the exclusion of philosophy from hermeneutics (which is based on the assumption that philosophical texts are rigorously conceptual rather than figurative in kind) would be untenable with regard to Hegel's thinking. Indeed Hegel's 'figures of speech' often provide essential guides to understanding his thinking.

Let us take a moment to consider what hermeneutics is. Recall that the modern term for the science of interpretation stems from the name of the Greek god, Hermes. Hermes is best known as the bearer of the messages of the gods to humans. But, lest we allow the honor of this post to bias our recollection of Hermes, let us also remember his characteristic habits and personality, which are of a considerably lower station. Hermes was a trickster and a theif. In the ancient Homeric hymns, the super-subtle Hermes is called "cattle-rustler", "carrier of dreams", "secret agent", "prowler."[63] A born liar, he invariably confused a message in conveying it, no matter how dire the situation. To his mother, Maia, he was a pain, sired by Zeus, she said, to be a headache to gods and men alike.[64]

The ancient portrayals of Hermes were perhaps the ways in which the Greeks fairly expressed the reigning confusion between gods and mortals (as well as misunderstandings between the gods themselves.) The ambiguity of the intentions of both immortals and mortals lies at the heart of Greek religion, art and politics. [65] For, as is witnessed by the pervasive practice of sacrifice in this culture, humans are forever making amends for having failed to hear the immortal decrees of the gods.

The most doubtful character of Hermes continued to play a role in the development and increasing importance of writing in classical Greek culture. For, as writing came to supplant the role of the oracle as the vehicle of universal truth in Greek society, understanding the gods and the lot of mortals become inextricably bound up with texts. One of the crucial transitions is of course the career of Socrates, who wrote not a word. But Plato was compelled to devote more attention to writing than to oracular speech, as indicated by his reflections on grammar (the art of writing) in the *Sophist*. By the time Aristotle gained ascendancy, writing had become a significant problem within philosophy.[66]

In the Hellenistic period, Western philosophy became embroiled in a bitter dispute spawned by Aristotle's philosophical understanding of writing. The tensions surrounding this concern became so great that Aristotle's academy split over it. Two major factions emerged in the centuries following Aristotle's death, one in the great center of learning, Alexandria, and the other in a less well-known center of learning, Pergamum. The schools were divided over whether grammar was more properly a science or an art. The Alexandrians pressed relentlessly to conceive of grammar as the science of constructing propositions. From this we have today the prescriptive grammar we all learned in school. The faction in Pergamum, on the other hand, presented grammar as the art of reading what has been handed down by tradition. From this developed the literary criticism which we practice today.[67]

Most of what characterizes modern hermeneutics stems from the Alexandrian, or scientific, conception of grammar. The task of writing is thought of as principally having to do with communicating one's thoughts on paper, and so the task of reading must be a matter of discerning the propositions as they were formed in the mind of the author. But "medieval" hermeneutics, as practiced in the period ranging from late Hellenistic times to the advent of modern hermeneutics at the turn of the eighteenth century, was quite different indeed. Less concerned with the author's original intentions in composing a given piece of writing, this hermeneutic focussed on the abiding meaning of texts. This model of reading stems from the 'artistic' school at Pergamum. It is still with us today (though it is under severe attack) in the practice of reading and interpreting the most influential texts of world literature. These 'classics' are read as crafted manipulations of perennial themes, problems, or lessons. They are interrogated for their abiding meanings.

The preeminent figure in the development of 'medieval' hermeneutics is Augustine of Hippo. For, in his *De Doctrina Christiana*, Augustine presents a general theory for reading texts which held from his day until modern times. His suggestion was to discover (especially through an elaborate use of analogy) one, singular message within the entire panoply of texts which at that time constituted the broad canon of Western culture. That message was the grace (*charitas*) of God.[68] But to accomplish such a vast re-reading involved reworking the original premise of hermeneutics. Hermes the trickster and befuddler, the vehicle of tragic misunderstanding, was replaced by Christ the savior his legion prophets, apostles, and disciples, the harbingers of true understanding. In short, the Christian Gospel, came to be held up as the paradigm for all of literature, whether it stemmed from the corpus of Biblical writings or the tradition of Classical culture.

With the coming of the Renaissance and early modernity, Augustine's hermenetics began slowly to unravel.[69] The general assumption, whether in its Greek or in its Christian form, that all texts convey knowledge of the divine was called into question. Methods of interpretation were developed to deal with texts as natural, or secular objects. The gradual rejection of the 'theological' hermeneutical assumption, and the refitting of hermeneutics for literary and legal texts became the basis for a hard-and-fast distinction between sacred and secular literature. The 'father' of this movement (not because he was the first, but because he became the most authoritative) was Friedrich Schleiermacher.

Schleiermacher's principal contribution to the history of hermeneutics was to argue, against the disintegrating tendencies of the modern critical attitude, that the problem of interpretation was universal. Thus all texts could be understood with the same method of reading. For each case of trying to discern the meaning of a given text (whether oral or written) was seen as a case of misunderstanding.

It is worth noting here that this starting point for interpretation draws more on the myth of Hermes the Trickster than on Christ as Savior. However, the system developed to solve the problem of misunderstanding could only be worked out by adopting certain assumptions which would dispell the myth of Hermes. For in the ancient scene the minds of the immortal gods were closed to all but Hermes. To think otherwise would be pure hubris. But Schleiermacher averred that the solution to the universal problem of interpretation was to assume the point of view of the author of the text in question. For, if one could know what the author was thinking, the meaning of the text would become clear.[70]

The consequence of this theory was to be the liberation of hermeneutics from the dogmatic assumptions of literary critics, legal scholars, and theologians. For, if the problem of interpretation was indeed universal, no special set of texts could be made to serve as the model for interpreting others (as had been the case in Augustine's hermeneutics), nor would the various types of specialized hermeneutics be divided with regard to method. Thus the universal nature of interpretation, which had indeed characterized medieval hermeneutics, was to be preserved, but the dogmatic adherence to certain theological texts was to be done away with. We have then a general science of interpretation which can explain sacred and secular texts alike.

However, as it turns out, Schleiermacher's 'universal' method of interpretation was in fact derived from his conception of theology.[71] And so, his hermeneutics ended up having much more in common with that of Augustine than he would have been ready to admit. It is just that with Schleiermacher, it was not the Gospel and its message of charity which served as the guide to interpretation, but rather the consciousness of God, or as he preferred, God-consciousness.[72] In short, by emphasizing that interpretation was always a form of misunderstanding, Schleiermacher was able to present a general hermeneutical principle which aided in undermining the dogmatic theology founded on the the inerrancy of Scripture and replacing it with a liberal theology rooted in self-awareness.[73]

Hegel, unlike Schleiermacher, did not develop a theory of interpretation. But, though he provided no general hermeneutics, he did present guidelines for reading the history of philosophy, and in connection with this, a general model for interpreting art, religion, and other cultural forms. Thus, while he may not be said to *have* a hermeneutical theory, he certainly employed a model of interpretation for coming to grips with the development of the Western tradition. A brief survey of the hermeneutical elements of Hegel's reading of philosophy will serve to introduce the particulars.

The method of reading philosophy employed in the *Differenzschrift* aims at understanding the relation of the finite and the infinite, appearance and the Absolute, the human and the divine. Thus, the reader of philosophy, like Hermes of old, announces the dictates of necessity. We understand by philosophy what is necessary, and such necessity explains the apparent world. And, like Augustine, Hegel seeks to discover one, singular meaning for all of the texts he has before his view. But, unlike Augustine, Hegel does not identify that meaning as the grace of God. Much rather it is the difference which lies at the heart of identity. While Augustine's hermeneutic is one of charity, Hegel's is one of fate, as we will see.

Other similarities between Augustine and Hegel are noteworthy in this context, most especially that both were concerned principally with the legacy of the written word. Art and religion bespeak the Absolute, even as philosophy does, for Hegel, but because philosophy is an exclusively written cultural form, it presents a different problem of interpretation than that found in art and religion. Philosophy, one might say, is a distinctly grammatical phenomenon. Art is part object, part speech, part writing. So too is religion.[74] But philosophy, Hegel reminds, dwells only within the written word, within systems. This basic distinction between philosophy as writing, and all other cultural forms accounts for the priority of philosophy over art and religion in Hegel's general notion of culture.[75] To the extent that the history of philosophy is bound within written texts, it is a radically hermeneutical affair: one can never appeal to the author's mind or intentions but only to the signs left to posterity.

Note also that both Augustine's and Hegel's concern with interpretation arose in response to a certain sort of cultural overload. When Augustine undertook to compose his manual of instruction for Christian instruction, it was during the time when Christianity had begun to develop as a world religion. This was due primarily to the fact that the Emperor Constantine had established the Christian faith as the official religion of the Roman Empire. The overnight success of Christianity led to grave problems. With the increase in status and prestige, the institution of Christianity had to come to grips with the fact that it was now a part of the Roman culture. Formerly it had been a provincial faith, competing with other such faiths. But now the world was its oyster, and so the history, literature, and science of the Greco-Roman world became the sometimes unruly charge of the Christian religion. Doubtless this strengthened the faith by rendering it more cosmopolitain and urbane, but it also threatened to destroy the integrity of the faith, to water it down.

Augustine's concern can be seen as the attempt to control the potentially damaging influence of non-Christian, non-theological texts and ideas, a threat which, incidentally, he knew well through his own experience as a professor of Classical rhetoric. He developed a general theory of interpretation to deal with the contingencies. He responded to the need of the times by showing how all words, no matter their source or manifest aim, signified the grace of God. Hegel, in his turn, proffered philosophy as the sole proper satisfaction for the need of his times. And, like Augustine, he accomplished this by developing a method of reading. Of course, the need of Hegel's day was not the same as that of Augustine's. It was not the prolific influence of Classical texts that Hegel fought against, though this did play a part in the drama, as we saw from his essay on excerpting. Rather Hegel struggled with the proliferation of philosophical opinions. This is where he decisively parts company with the Augustinian tradition.

Hegel was of a mind that the integrity of philosophy had been seriously, even mortally, weakened by relativism. It seemed that there were as many private truths as there were philosophers. The only consensus of the day seemed to be that philosophy was a matter of personal opinion. This assumption worried Hegel deeply. He demanded, against the indifference of the times, that there was but one true philosophy. He averred that all philosophical texts conspire, more or less, to utter one unique meaning, namely, the appearance of the Absolute, or Reason, as he sometimes preferred to call it. It might be added that it did not matter whether the texts in question were ancient, contemporary, dogmatic, common sensical, critical, or speculative. It did not matter whether they were axiomatic treatises on philosophy, as were Spinoza's writings, or personal reflections on philosophical themes, as were Pascal's *Pensees*. It did not matter whether they were written in Greek, Latin, French, English, or German.[76] Finally, and most emphatically, it did not matter one iota what the authors had in mind in committing their words to paper, nor what others had thought upon reading them. The only issue of any real import was what the text said for or against the Absolute. But by what means could Hegel justify such an imperial practice of reading?

By way of explanation, let us return to the issue of the need of philosophy. Recall that, according to Hegel's view, the development of philosophy in the modern period had led to the rigid fixation of opposites into dichotomies. Philosophy had painted itself into a corner, as it were, and matters appeared hopeless. One by one philosophers had thrown up their hands in defeat. Truth had been abandoned by the ranks, and the end of philosophy was at hand. Hegel's response was to argue, quite strenuously, that this had not merely happened; it was necessary. His response was in part unoriginal. For Kant had already established in his first *Critique* a dialectic of reason which resultued in certain inevitable antinomies. And to this extent, we should not blame Hegel for coming up with an uncharitable reading of the history of philosophy. What was original in his response, however, was his claim that the dialectic of reason was but a failed form of speculative philosophy, that the history of philosophical failures was in fact but one side of the matter. What needed to be established was the turn from the oppositions of the understanding to the identity and difference of thinking. He was therefore at pains to show that the many errors which made up the history of philosophy had something in common, something which could bring about a solution to the difficulties at hand and bring a renewed vitality to philosophy.

The proof of his claim was provided by applying the cardinal principle of his philosophical hermeneutic: Every philosophy is complete in itself, and like an authentic work of art, carries the totality within itself. But, we might wonder, if this is indeed the case, why must it be emphatically pressed upon us? Why can we not anticipate this and so avoid the pitfall of fragmented understanding. It is because, "In [any] culture, the appearance of the Absolute has become isolated from the Absolute and fixated into independece." This is the fate of philosophy. What is in truth one appears as divided; division becomes dichotomy; people take up sides, and so dissension ultimately reigns.

The second principle of Hegel's hermeneutic is that there is no way to bridge the gap between the Absolute and its appearance. The history of philosophy is the attempt to do just this, but it is a failed attempt, because rather than constructing a bridge, it has managed only to erect a museum, and then fill it with the pet opinions of famous philosophers. This is because philosophy has become fixated on appearance, dividing it into pairs or opposites, antinomies, and the like. Hence like, a Kafkaesque castle, the house of philosophy is a labyrinth. Whenever the understanding comes up against something other than itself, it draws a distinction, creating a wall. Then it divides the wall, or rather outlines a door through the wall, and so creates another partition within knowledge. Distinction after distinction, door after door, until finally one gives up, and decides to live within the compartment of one's own making. Thus there is no way out of this philosophical penal colony. Save one. The edifice of philosophy must be razed to the ground. But how?

Hegel's suggestion is perhaps too easy to seem plausible. It is to let thought think itself. Not to let thought think an object, but to turn thinking upon itself in a reflexive form. This is what we examined before under the name of speculation: Speculation is the one universal Reason directed upon itself. How, though, is this to be accomplished in general? Paradoxically, it might seem, by giving up. Not by giving up thinking, but by giving up one's thoughts, one's opinions:

> The essence of philosophy ... is a bottomless abyss for personal idiosyncrasy. In order to reach philosophy it is necessary to throw oneself into it *a corps perdu*—meaning by 'body' here, the sum of one's idiosyncrasies. (Ibid., p. 88)

To do philosophy, then, is not to think thoughts, but to 'go under' as it were, to undertake an initiatic death, whereby one lets go of whatever one thought was the truth.[77] This is to pursue philosophy, as Hegel puts it, without presupposiitons. And is this not the meaning of Socrates's ignorance? Did not Descartes begin with radical, absolute doubt?

Hegel maintains that in thus 'opening' one's mind, the philosopher will come to realize that he is not alone. Indeed he will discern his true affinity with others who have done likewise:

> The particular speculative Reason [of a later time] finds in [its age] spirit of its spirit, flesh of its flesh, it intuits itself in it as one and the same and yet as another living being. (Ibid.)

Here the initiatic death of philosophy grants a new sense of life, a life for the first time worth living. It also grants philosophy a future.

Let us not make the mistake of thinking that Hegel's writings are the last word in philosophy. Rather they are the occasion for philosophy, in his life, and, by way of example, in the lives of others. Philosophy will be carried on by writing, or the system of discourse. No such system will be able to reach full closure, inasmuch as it is recognized as the appearance of the Absolute, rather than the Absolute itself. But this can only be made intelligle and constructive by knowing that the need of philosophy is in its core a hermeneutical need. It involves the never-ending process of construing the parts of philosophy in relation to a whole known only intuitively. This is not to deny that there is a whole, only that the whole is exhausted by any of its appearances. This is also to say that the whole is not known, save through its parts, and then only incompletely, or hermeneutically.

To the extent that Hegel was successful in his attempt at reading philosophy, the character of philosophy changed. That change involves a certain sort of liberation. Hegel's philosophical hermeneutic frees the reader from the manifold opinions of philosophers not by merely leveling the genuine differences between philosophical systems, but by identifying the individuality of those systems as various forms of perennial wisdom. Thus in the *Differenzschrift* Hegel painstakingly differentiates the subjective idealism of Fichte from the objective idealism of Schelling in order to allow the reader to apprehend both as forms of thought thinking itself. And by showing that thought can think itself in at least two different ways, he has demonstrated conclusively that different philosophical systems are not mere differences of opinion. Thus philosophy is saved from dead opinion and liberated for life.

It is important to note, however, that this is not all Hegel accomplished in his *Differenzschrift*. He also realized that he might well be able to compose a philosophical system himself, one which would differ significantly from those of his predecessors and contemporaries, without being guilty of merely adding another room on to the philosophical prison house of opinion. His hermeneutic granted him the freedom to value his own individuality as a philosopher. It signaled a coming of age. And so, at the end of the long essay, he was able to allude genuinely and sincerely to his designs on a speculative system which would soon be launched in his contributions to the *Critical Journal of Philosophy*.

Perhaps the most significant aspect of Hegel's newfound philosophical freedom was that he recognized that dialectic, the drawing of distinctions, could indeed be genuinely speculative[78]—that even in working out the differences which made up the philosophy of his day, he could rise above it by articulating the origin and end of philosophy itself.[79] With this realization came a confidence in language. Language could be made to speak speculatively, and not merely argumentatively. Writing could become the form and substance of a philosophical system. He had tapped into the *logos* of thinking without become entrapped in the formal dogmatic structures of grammar and logic and lexicon.

I identified the cardinal principle of Hegel's philosophical hermeneutic above to be that each philosophy is complete in itself, like a work of art. What needs to be added to this is the philosophical insight which this principle expresses. For Hegel did not merely borrow an aesthetic principle and naively apply it to philosophy. His understanding of art is based on his conception of philosophy, as is apparent from what he says in the *Differenzschrift* about the relation of art, religion, and philosophy as cultural forms. That conception, as we have noted above, is without presupposition, without a higher ground. What we might be inclined to call the presupposition of philosophy, recall, is what Hegel deemed the utterance of the need of philosophy. As we have learned to recognize, that need, in its necessary form, is dichotomy. It is this dichotomy which finds its adequate expression in speculative discourse. That discourse, as was argued in Chapter One, is paradigmatically present in the utterance of the death of God.

It might seem a bit of a stretch to say that, because every philosophy carries totality within it, this phrase itself can bear the full burden of philosophy. But if we recognize that, for Hegel, philosophy always appears in the form of a system, and that his system in particular appears as speculative discourse, and further that speculative discourse has its paradigm in the phrase, God is dead, then it is not incorrect to claim that this phrase is the appearance of totality. In this we see that Hegel's philosophical hermenetic is at work, not only in his reading of philosophy, but in the generation of his own philosophical system.

Speculation and Common Sense

Let us now turn to Hegel's dicussion of the relation of speculation to common sense to see how he put his hermeneutic principles to work in bringing learning in line with life.

In speculation the piecemeal elements of everyday knowledge, known as common sense, are subsumed under the totality of the Absolute.[80] But, if the conventional wisdom of common sense provides us with practical guides for life, still practical knowledge as such has no real standing, and so cannot constitute learning itself. The pitfall of common sense, according to Hegel, lies in taking its half-truths as genuine knowledge. These truths cannot be adequately expressed, save by speculation, whereby they are placed in relation to the Absolute. But, though it is clear to speculation that the truths of common sense have their standing only in the Absolute, common sense is blind to the work of speculation. Thus, in the task of bringing learning to life, speculation is opposed by common sense.

Speculation, however, cannot leave the truths of common sense aside, no matter the "hatred and persecution" it meets.[81] For speculation, if it is to be the expression of learning in its essential relation to life, must display common sense's immediate grasp, its certainty, of reality as the dim apprehension of the Absolute. To this end, Hegel distinguishes between the unconscious, or pre-reflective, grasp of truth in common sense and the post-conscious, or post-reflective, grasp of the truth in speculation.[82] The difference between the two is entrenched in what he calls faith.[83]

As a product of *Reflexion*, faith sunders the identity of the relative and the Absolute, common sense and speculative reason. But the immediate certitude of faith proper to common sense really belongs to reason, though only unconsciously so. Because common sense does not recognize reason in its faith, it opposes speculation.[84] But, Hegel presses, common sense and speculation can and should unite.[85] This meeting, however, can only occur if reason sunders itself. For the destruction of *Reflexion*, the irradication of faith, is the submission of Absolute identity, played out in the sphere of reason:

> Reason thus drowns itself and its knowledge and its reflection of the absolute identity, in its own abyss: and in this night of mere reflection and of the calculating intellect, in this night which is the noonday of life, common sense and speculation can meet one another." (Ibid., p. 103)

As such the meeting of common sense and speculation under the glare of a post-reflective noon-day sun is the point of departure for philosophy proper.

Philosophy as System

The final section of the introduction, entitled *Relation of Philosophizing to a Philosophical System*, returns to the notion of the need of philosophy.[86] Here Hegel maintains that the need of philosophy can be met by rooting out faith, and uniting common sense with speculation.[87] Only when the piecemeal apprehension of ordinary truths is taken in its connection with the whole of the Absolute, is the need of philosophy truly satisfied. This is an important point, for otherwise, one might think that philosophy could take the mystical form of silently beholding the coincidence of opposites. But this would be to give up on the task of bringing learning to life. For Hegel, the apprehension of this coincidence does not and cannot remain silent. It must be brought to speech. It must be articulated. For it is the voice of spirit expressed in living language, in language tied to culture.

Yet once the Absolute is uttered, it is bound up with the problem of interpretation. Words ever say more and less than we mean. They outstrip our intentions, and so we cannot hold our thoughts fast. Heraclitus expressed this in saying that one cannot step into the same river twice. Hegel's response is to radicalize this insight: one cannot step into the same river even once. For sameness (identity) involves self-relation (difference.) Thus thinking, even consciousness in general, must come to grips with the problem of recollecting the parts into a whole.[88]

The hermeneutical need of philosophy demands that the part be taken in relation to the whole, but it also grants that the need of philosophy can be met even when the parts are not presented in their interconnection.[89] Hegel's conception of the relation of the part and the whole, therefore, implies that the need of philosophy can be met in part: the part can by itself be conceived as the appearance of the whole. But, so long as the part is taken in isolation from other such parts, the Absolute cannot be manifest as an objective totality:

> Since the finite things are a manifold, the connection of the finite to the
> Absolute is a manifold. Hence, philosophizing must aim to posit this
> manifold as internally connected, and there necessarily arises the need
> to produce a totality of knowing, a system of science. (Ibid., p. 113)

Yet when the manifold of particulars is articulated in an objective totality of knowledge, the need of philosophy is wholly met.

The articulation of the manifold of particulars in an objective totality of knowledge, i.e., in a system, is, according to Hegel, the work of speculative reason.[90] However, any such totality has only a relative identity to the Absolute.[91] A system of philosophy is a duplicate[92] of the Absolute identity of the whole and the sum of its parts. Accordingly, no system can be the Absolute. Because the Absolute and philosophical systems are not co-extensive, the need of philosophy is finally a hermeneutical need:

> The history of philosophy only has value and interest if it holds fast to
> this viewpoint. For otherwise, it will not give us the history of the one,
> eternal Reason, presenting itself in infinitely manifold forms; instead it
> will give us nothing but a tale of the accidental vicissitudes of the human
> spirit and of senseless opinions, which the teller imputes to Reason,
> though they should be laid only on to his own charge, because he does
> not recognize what is rational in them, and so turns them inside out.

Hegel's essay proceeds from this point to consider its proper subject, namely, the relation of the systems of Fichte and Schelling. His exposition is an example of the hermeneutical principle outlined above, and so can be recounted here in cursory fashion: Fichte's philosophy presents a system of knowledge which is based upon the relative, subjective identity of subject and object, and so it presupposes but does not articulate speculation. Schelling's philosophy, on the other hand, propounds a system of knowledge which embodies the absolute identity of subject and object, and is therefore an adequate expression of philosophy.[93]

The Hermeneutical Absolute

Before leaving this work, however, we might summarize our findings with regard to Hegel's notion of philosophy. Speculation, he avers, always begins properly with the absolute identity of subject and object. But, because the Absolute sunders itself, manifesting itself in the dichotomy between subject and object, speculation must become critical. For it must now deal with the appearance of the Absolute, rather than the Absolute in-itself. Criticism is the apprehension of the Absolute in its contingent forms. But, as such, criticism must become speculative.

Otherwise it will lose itself in appearance, either mistaking the knowledge of appearance for philosophy itself, as did Kant, or by denying the knowledge of appearance and so philosophy itself, as did the "scepticism"[94] of Hegel's day. Thus, if criticism is to hold fast to appearance as appearance, it must return to speculation, the basis of the distinction between appearance and the Absolute itself. But now the task of speculation has been altered. The Absolute, its starting point, must now be discovered as the result of speculation. The hermeneutical principle which guides speculation at this point is that the Absolute is to be discovered amidst appearance as the manifestation of the Absolute in relative form; that the part is the manifestation of a whole comprising more than the mere sum of its parts.

In the *Critical Journal of Philosophy* we will see Hegel take up the speculative-critical task of discerning the whole in the parts of the philosophy of his day and of construing the whole which is the sum of those parts. In particular we will see Hegel following a course of criticism that leads his reader to a crisis in faith and philosophy, a crisis wherein the Absolute is manifest in the feeling that "God Himself is dead." But we will also see Hegel lead his reader beyond this crisis, to speculatively utter the death of God. For a speculative-critical grasp of the death of God is at once the end of philosophizing (i.e., opinionizing) and the beginning of philosophy proper (i.e., speculative discourse). Finally we will see Hegel put his speculative philosophy to work in a reconsideration of the matter of freedom and necessity from the perspective of the death of God.

ENDNOTES

[1]Hegel did not use the term relativism. As we will learn in Chapter Four, he identified the culprit as dogmatic scepticism.

[2]Johann Wolfgang von Goethe, *Faust*, trans. Charles E. Passage, The Library of Liberal Arts (Indianapolis: The Bobbs-Merrill Company, 1965.)

[3]Harris notes that Hegel probably first began to take the philosophy of identity seriously when he and Hölderlin labored in Frankfurt (1795) to discover a "higher synthesis" for the division between Spinoza's philosophy of nature and Fichte's philosophy of freedom. Needless to say, he found himself in good company with Schelling in Jena, for Schelling had by then become the leading proponent of the *Identitätsphilosophie*. See Diff., p. 3ff.

[4]SW Vol. 1, pp. 31-168.

[5]Harris comments in his introduction to the *Differenzschrift* that this essay represents the "...first chapter of a 'discourse on method' which Hegel carried on for the rest of his life." See Diff. p. 15.

[6]Though Harris makes no explicit reference to the question of hermeneutics in his introduction to this piece, he brings the matter to light in an interesting way by remarking that, for Hegel, "...nothing contains its own explanation within itself, nothing is its own *logos*." See ibid. p. 29. Harris's comment is made in the context of a discussion of Hegel's criticism of the notion of

causality, but I think it is not to stretch matters too far to suggest that, for Hegel, causation is a form of explanation, and hence in a certain sense a hermeneutical concern. Surely Nietzsche's Will to Power as interpretation and Heidegger's ontology is in keeping with this insight.

[7]Ibid. p. 18.

[8]Ibid. p. xii.

[9]Ibid. p. 83. The translators note that Hegel is here referring generally to the *Critical Journal of Philosophy* and more specifically to the article, *Faith and Knowledge*.

[10]Ibid. p. 195.

[11]See Buchner and Pöggeler in the appendix to GW Vol IV, p. 534.

[12]For the complete text see Ros., pp. 448-51.

[13]Ibid. pp. 454-458.

[14]Ibid. p. 10. See also GB p. 14f and Sunlight, p. 3f.

[15]I refer here principally to the material compiled in the *Early Theological Writings*. Richard Kroner, in his introduction to the English translation of this work, describes Hegel's attitude toward traditional religious authority as follows:

> "Religion, he then held, should not be learned from books or confined to dogma, memory, and moral rules; it should not be a theological religion. Rather it should be a living power, flourishing in the real life of a nation, in their habits, ideals, customs, actions, and festivals, in their hearts and will, in their deeds as well as in their imagination." (*Early Theological Writings*, p. 3f.)

It might be noted in passing that Kroner's comment suggests that Hegel's interest in a tolerant attitude toward religion is not so much rooted in the rationalism of the Enlightenment tradition of natural religion, as in the sensibility of Romantic thought. On this matter see Sunlight, p. 6. Harris holds that the Enlightenment tradition upon which Hegel drew early on was that which carried forward the cause of Renaissance humanism. But this suggestion must be tempered by the fact of Kant's influence upon Hegel at this time, for Hegel did not uncritically accept the positivity of religion. See *Early Theological Writings*, p. 4ff and Sunlight p. 34 footnote 1.

[16]Just why Hegel chose philosophy over religion at this stage is a matter of considerable concern which must be closely attended in the discussion to follow.

[17]For other accounts, see Walter Cerf's general introduction in Diff. Also of help are Mark C. Taylor, *Disfiguring*, p. 40f. and William Desmond, *Beyond Hegel and Dialectic, passim*.

[18]Hegel does not employ the term, nihilism, in the *Differenzschrift*, but he does in the article on faith and knowledge. There he speaks of a latent nihilism in the philosophy of Kant, and more especially, of Fichte. See Faith, p. 168ff.

[19]This important point will be treated in detail in subsequent analysis of the *Differenzschrift*.

[20]Just why this occasion is superficial will become apparent in what follows.

[21]Cerf and Harris note the following in their translation: Reinhold believed the revolution was accomplished in the work of C.G. Bardili, *Grundriss der Ersten Logik* (Stuttgart, 1800). The full title of this work was: *"Outline of Primary Logic* purified from the errors of previous Logics generally, and of the Kantian logic in particular; not a Critique but a *medicina mentis*, to be employed mainly for Germany's Critical Philosophy." See Diff., p. 79, footnote 3.

[22]See SW Vol. 1, p. 33f. The reference here is to Kant's *Critique of Pure Reason*, especially Chapter Two of the Transcendental Analytic.

[23]SW Vol. 1, p. 34.

[24]Cerf and Harris note that Hegel here refers to Kant's *Critique of Judgement*. See Diff., p. 81.

[25]See SW Vol. 1, p. 34f.

[26]Fichte's claim that this principle is the basis of the Kantian philosophy is to be found in the second introduction to the *Science of Knowledge.* See Cerf and Harris Diff., p. 79.

[27]SW Vol. 1, p. 35.

[28]Hegel's point relies upon reading "*sollen*" as a subjunctive (i.e., a condition contrary to fact), rather than as an imperative. Thus to say that something "ought" to be such and so, connotes that it "is" not so.

[29]Ibid. p. 35f.

[30]Ibid. 36.

[31]Ibid. p. 40. Charles Taylor sounds this theme in his commentary on Hegel's *History of Philosophy.* He remarks that philosophy "comes after life" and that it is an unusual sort of cultural form because of its "tardy appearance and recapitulative role." See *Hegel* (Cambridge University Press, 1975) p. 511. I might add that it is true in a sense that philosophy is afterthought, and as such it involves recollection (*Erinnerung.*) But to say that it is always too late is to go too far. We will see that Hegel develops a notion of philosophy in which afterthought is itself generative, or original. Recollection in this sense is not a remembrance of things past, but an evocation of the present. This is no where more clear than in Hegel's notion of the history of philosophy as the appearance of the eternal in the present.

[32]See SW Vol. 1 p. 39f.

[33]Ibid.

[34] I assume that the "living spirit" and the Absolute are synonymous here.

[35]It should be noted that Hegel holds that both the Absolute and its appearance, reason, are eternal. It is in its eternity that reason is the essence of philosophy.

[36]Ibid. p. 41.

[37]Surely Hegel is here alluding to the following passage from Kant's First Critique:

> "We have now not merely explored the territory of pure understanding, and carefully surveyed every part of it, but have also measured its extent, and assigned to everything in it its rightful place. This domain is an island, enclosed by nature itself within unalterable limits. It is the land of truth—enchanting name!—surrounded by a wide and stormy ocean, the native home of illusion, where many a fog bank and many a swiftly melting iceberg give the deceptive appearance of farther shores, deluding the adventurous seafarer ever anew with empty hopes, and engaging him in enterprises which he can never abandon and yet is unable to carry to completion."
> See CPR p. 257.

[38]This is not, as Cerf maintains (see Diff., p. xxi), a matter of the "resurrection" of philosophy. Rather opinion must die so that thought can live.

[39]Cerf puts it well:

> "In a very preliminary way we can describe what the author of the *Essays* [i.e. the contents of the *Critical Journal of Philosophy* attributable to Hegel] meant by speculation as the intuition or vision of the true nature of the relations among God, nature, and self-consciousness or reason." (Diff., p. xi)

[40]SW Vol. 1, p. 43.

[41]Again the question arises as to why Hegel holds that philosophy is to be the point of departure for speculation, rather than poetry, art, religion, or history, for example. Our question and his

answer, however, are only implicit in his essay, and so must be allowed to develop as the discussion advances.

[42]See Harris's note in Diff., p. 89.

[43]SW Vol. 1 p. 37.

[44]See Diff., p. 91.

[45]Hegel's point seems to be that, once art has been sundered in the forms of fetishism and fantasy, the self-consciously imaginative element of religion and the gravity of play are suppressed. The twofold result is magic and mimicry, both of which lack an essential connection to culture as the balance of life and learning. This failure of art originally occured, according to Hegel, in classical Greece, "long ago and far away." See ibid.

[46]This is a difficult passage. Hegel presents the notion of a determinate religion as an example, perhaps a paradigmatic one, of the highest aesthetic fulfillment. He says that humankind transcends the division of culture in this form. But he seems also to say that the essential opposition of subject and object remains in the notion of the kingdom of grace. Thus, while a determinate religion presents the possibility of overcoming all forms of the division of culture hitherto, it fails precisely at the point of resolving the opposition of subject and object; the kingdom of grace thus intensifies the latest and most virulent form of division, namely, that of the opposition of subject and object in the philosophy of reflection. Religion, therefore, would be seen to stand between art and philosophy, when matters are considered according to their contingency, but would be identified with the philosophy of reflection, as regards necessity. This failure of culture occured, in Hegel's account, with the Reformation. See ibid.

[47]The reference here is to Descartes. See ibid.

[48]It should be noted that, though this stage marks the appearance of necessity, still it is only the penultimate stage in the full development of culture. The ultimate stage is that wherein philosophy proper emerges from out of religion and the philosophy of reflection. At this point it becomes manifest that the contingent cultural progression from art to religion finds its necessity in philosophy. Accordingly, the significance of art for religion and *vice versa*, which was obscured by the understanding, becomes clear. This much is manifest in the *Phenomenology*'s discussion of art and religion which has its philosophical epicenter in the notion of the religion of art. See PG pp. 535-569. This point was also made in Chapter One of the present investigation.

[49]SW Vol. 1 p. 44f. The metaphor here need not be a biblical one. Hegel's allusion could as easily be to Plato's Cave, which philosophy posits as the abode of the understanding. The shadow world within the Cave corresponds to the world of appearance lying between human understanding and the Absolute truth of the sun. So long as philosophy dwells within the cave, attempting to interpret the play of shadows, it confines itself to a manifold which is in truth only a part of the genuine whole constituted by the sun and all upon which it shines. Harris, for example, takes the Platonic metaphor of the Cave as a fruitful vehicle for understanding Hegel's early philosophical development. See Sunlight, p. xxxii. Harris fails to take the crucial step, however, of identifying the sun not with reason, but with speculative insight, as discussed above. For only when the sun is seen as the speculum of thinking, does the philosopher discover reason therein. Hegel's dissertation on the solar system and his comments in the *Critical Journal of Philosophy* regarding Krug's superficial understanding of the sun indicate this. This topic will surface again in Chapter Four.

[50]SW Vol. 1 p. 45. Perhaps here more than anywhere else it is clear that Hegel is referring to the philosophical system of Kant. For in that system is to be found the high water mark of the philosophical tide of understanding. That the emergence of the Kantian philosophy on the cultural scene was contemporaneous with the outbreak of the French Revolution, and the general restlessness of the age further supports Hegel's insight into the relation between philosophy and culture.

[51]It should be noted here that the Hegelian opposite of negation is not affirmation, but the identity of positing and negating, namely, the Absolute.

[52]Hegel's proposition is the following:

> "In the infinite activity of becoming and producing, Reason has united what was sundered and it has reduced the absolute dichotomy to a relative one, one that is conditioned by the original identity." (Diff., p. 91)

To take up philosophy as reason is to conceive of its internal opposition between subject and object as the necessary division of an original identity, namely the Absolute.

[53]Unfortunately there is no other way to express it. Yet the notion of a return should not be conceived as the simple re-enstatement of a previous state of affairs. As with the old saw, that one cannot go home again, reason returns to the Absolute, but reason has changed in the interim. This point will be taken up later, in its proper context.

[54]Another main tenet of Hegel's thinking finds expression here. The production, or discovery, of the Absolute by reason presupposes that the Absolute goes out of itself, articulating a course that can be navigated by reason. In this respect the *Logic* is the presupposition of the *Phenomenology*. See SW Vol. 4, p. 43f. This point has also been discussed in my introduction.

[55]Ibid. p. 48. The preposition, *in*, here takes the accusative case, and thus denotes a passage from the finite into the infinite rather than a positing of the finite within the infinite.

[56]A final note in passing regarding the relation of the *Phenomenology* and the *Logic-Encyclopaedia*. If the former can be identified with the night and the latter with the day, then life is the union of appearance and becoming. And, if the task of philosophy is to enliven learning, then philosophy is expressed in Hegel's thought in the union of the *Phenomenology* and the *Logic-Encyclopaedia*. This is by way of suggesting that Hegel's thought consists in suspending the absolute difference between his two greatest works.

[57]My way of putting matters implies an important distinction between reflection as such and understanding. The distinction is Hegel's, and it is expressed in his formulation, to be considered below, of *Reflexion als Vernunft*. To the extent that reflection can be seen as reason, it is not identical with understanding. For reason and understanding are mutually exclusive in Hegel's scheme. However, reflection also appears, according to Hegel, in the form of the understanding. Thus, if reflection is at once reason and understanding, it must have within it a basic division. This division is apparent in the German *Reflexion*. *Reflexion* denotes, on one hand, the relation of subject and object, as considered from the perspective of subjectivity. This is the sense of the English term, reflection; the subject reflects upon an object, and hence the object is the reflection (image) of subjectivity. On the other hand, *Reflexion* denotes the relation of subject and object, as viewed from the "point of indifference" between the two. This sense is not conveyed by the English; *Reflexion* is the double relation of subject and object, their conditioning of one another. In the former sense, *Reflexion* is associated with the subjective faculty of the understanding. In the latter sense, it is connected with reason. I will henceforth employ *Reflexion* in order to preserve its technical usage in Hegel's discussion.

[58]Ibid. p. 50.

[59]Hegel's reasoning is based upon the basic tenet that the Absolute is not merely something posited or determinate. But to limit it, or to pose it as a limit, is to render it determinate, positive.

[60]Ibid. p. 51.

[61]The metaphor of a battle between reason and understanding has now reverted to a struggle within *Reflexion* itself. Just as in the nautical metaphor Hegel employed above, the danger faced by philosophy as understanding is nothing to philosophy as reason. Inasmuch as *Reflexion*,

as the instrument of philosophizing, identifies itself with understanding, it must destroy itself. But in the self-destruction of the understanding, *Reflexion* attains its genuine standing in the Absolute.

[62]Ibid. p. 54.

[63]*The Homeric Hymns,* trans. by Charles Boer, 2nd edition (Dallas, Texas: Spring Publications, Inc., 1970) p. 18.

[64]Ibid. p. 29.

[65]This fact made a distinct impression on Hegel, as we have noted above, for his interest in classical drama, e.g., Sophocles's *Antigone* and Aeschylus's *Eumenides*, as well as his respect for Goethe's *Iphigenia*, was rooted in the "ambiguity" which drives the plot in these tragedies.

[66]For a brief and informative discussion of this topic see Martin Heidegger, *An Introduction to Metaphysics,* trans. by Ralph Manheim (Garden City, New York: Doubleday & Company, Inc., 1961) p. 47f.

[67]An informative account of this development is to be found in Rudolf T. Schmidt, *Die Grammatik der Stoiker,* intro. by K. Hülser (Braunschweig; Wiesbaden; Vieweg, 1979) pp. 9-14.

[68]For a succinct discussion of Augustine's contribution to reading the canon of Western literature see Robertson's introduction in *On Christian Doctrine,* trans. by D.W. Robertson, Jr. (Indianapolis: The Bobbs-Merrill Company, Inc., 1978) pp. x-xi. The basic premise of Augustine's hermeneutic is as follows, "[E]very good and true Christian should understand that wherever he may find truth, it is his Lord's." (p. 54)

[69]The new science of early modernity tended to be critical of the received wisdom of the Church. This new attitude toward knowledge employed Augustinian techniques of interpretation even as it worked against the premise of Augustine's method. The seeds of this critical method were sown by such figures as Petrarch and Lorenzo Valla. The rise of textual criticism in early modernity is briefly outlined in W. T. Jones, *A History of Western Philosophy: Hobbes to Hume,* second edition (HBJ, 1969) pp. 36ff.

[70]Debates have raged over this issue in recent years. It was long held that Schleiermacher appealed to a form of divination whereby the interpreter projected himself into the mind of the author in order to understand his words. Lately scholars of Schleiermacher have sought to debunk this position by pointing out that his interest was not with the intention of the author, but with the authorial point of view. This distinction is subtle but important for the task of interpretation. For it emphasizes that there is no access to the author, save through the words of the text. But, as we will see, this insight was probably not true of Schleiermacher's hermeneutics. On this subject see Hans-Georg Gadamer, *Truth and Method* (New York: Crossroad Publishing Company, 1975) pp. 157-173.

[71]For Gadamer's assessment of this matter see ibid., p. 173.

[72]For Schleiermacher's notion of God-consciousness see his *The Christian Faith,* ed. by H.R. Mackintosh and J.S. Stewart (Edinburgh: T&T Clark, 1986) pp. 131-141.

[73]It is because of this shift from the authority of the Bible to the authority of consciousness that Schleiermacher is recognized as the founder of modern theology.

[74]This is to anticipate the perspective of the *Phenomenology,* where religion is ultimately a form of art.

[75]Derrida has made this point, rather cryptically, in his assessment of Hegel as the "last philosopher of the book, and the first thinker of writing." See *Of Grammatology,* trans. by Gayatri Chakravorty Spivak (Baltimore: Johns Hopkins University Press, 1980) p. 26.

[76]German, of course, presents a problem here, for as we have seen Hegel maintained that his mother tongue had a certain priority over other languages with respect to philosophy.

[77]We saw the corollary of this in the preceding explication of speculation. For, recall that one cannot properly see oneself in the speculum of the eye. The focus on oneself must of necessity be abandoned in the insight into speculation.

[78]Gadamer sheds important light on this topic in his discussion of Hegel's dialectic. The gist of his comments is that "Hegel's dialectic ... follows the speculative spirit of language ..." See op. cit., p. 426. But for the broader context of Gadamer's analysis, in which he indicates the limitations of Hegel's dialectic for the problem of hermeneutics, see ibid. pp. 414-431. The focus of the present study does not permit me to refute Gadamer's assertion that Hegel's speculative philosophy does not "attain to the linguistic experience of the world." But from what I have said about the role of language in Hegel's philosophy, it should be apparent that I cannot accept Gadamer's assessment.

[79]Goethe has provided a fine example of this transcendence in an example drawn from the natural world: "In many of its tones the nightingale is only a bird; then it rises up above its class, and seems as if it would teach every feathered creature what singing really is." From *Elective Affinities*, trans. by James Anthony Froude and R. Dillon Boylan (Frederick Ungar Publishing, Co. 1977) p. 203.

[80]SW Vol. 1 p. 55.

[81]Ibid. p. 56f.

[82]I employ the terminology of pre- and post-reflective truth here to emphasize Hegel's positioning of reflection between common sense and speculation.

[83]Ibid. p. 57.

[84]Ibid. p. 57f.

[85]Ibid. p. 60.

[86]I skip over the intervening sections, since they explicate in further detail the basic problem of the philosophy of reflection in relation to the notion of intellectual intuition implicit in Hegel's conception of speculation.

[87]Ibid. p. 70.

[88]The problem of recollection (*Erinnerung*) becomes thematic in the *Phenomenology*.

[89]Ibid. p. 71.

[90]Ibid. p. 71f.

[91]As will be seen in the passage to follow, Hegel also refers to this as a subjective identity, or as self-consciousness.

[92]It should be noted that Hegel's term *Duplicität* is problematic. Absolute identity is the identity of subject and object. The relative identity in question, however, is only the identity of part and whole which prevails in subjectivity, namely, self-consciousness. The difference between the two is expressed in Hegel's claim that absolute identity is conditioned by its "duplicate" relative identity. When absolute identity is thought as conditioned by relative identity, dogmatism results. (Ibid. p. 72) In this respect the relation of the two identities is duplicitous. Thus the need for a system of knowledge is the need of absolute identity to be freed from the contingency of its appearance in the relative identity, of philosophy to be freed from dogmatism, of the truth to be freed from duplicity. However, once the subjectivity of self-consciousness has been identified with the objective totality of knowledge, absolute identity is manifest as it truly is in itself.

[93]It should be pointed out here that Hegel gives Schelling more credit than he perhaps deserves. For, as Harris points out, Schelling had not yet produced a system of philosophy as such. Later in his life, Hegel conceded this. See Diff., p. 7. The fact that Hegel saw more in Schelling's writings than did others suggests that he already saw beyond the limitations of his friend's thought.

[94]Hegel pursues this topic in an article on scepticism, to be considered in detail in Chapter Four.

PART TWO: THE CRITICAL JOURNAL OF PHILOSOPHY

The setting for Hegel's utterance of the death of God is the Critical Journal of Philosophy (1802-03). The substance of what he wrote regarding the history of philosophy in his contributions to this journal provides a developed sketch of his emergent system. In this part of our investigation, we will expose the death of God as the epicenter of Hegel's contributions to this journal. We will proceed with an exposition of the full written context of Hegel's utterance.

4

CRITICISM, COMMON SENSE AND SCEPTICISM.

In 1801 Hegel began to publish his endeavors in systematic philosophy. Whether because of a lack of confidence or because the occasion was not right, he did not pursue his system openly. More likely even is the possibility that he felt the need to know more before he displayed his first attempt at a system of thought. In any case, he continued in the vein of the *Differenzschrift* to speak in the third person, as a critic of philosophy and culture, rather than as a contributor. Nevertheless, as we will see in his publications in the *Critical Journal of Philosophy*, he had indeed already begun to sketch in the basic outlines of his original philosophical program.

Let us now turn to the *Critical Journal* itself to see the development of Hegel's early publications. Co-authored by Hegel and Schelling, the journal ran two years, comprising six issues. To show their unity of purpose and mind in this enterprise, the two writers refrained from claiming authorship for any of the individual articles.[1]

This raises the question of authorship in the case of each of the several articles contained in the journal. There is a long history of disputes over the authorship of given articles that goes back to Hegel and Schelling themselves.[2] As matters stand presently, a consensus has been reached that the following articles belong without a reasonable doubt to Hegel: "*Ueber das Wesen der philosophischen Kritik überhaupt, und ihr Verhältniss zum gegenwärtigen Zustand der Philosophie insbesondere,*" "*Wie der gemeine Menschenverstand die Philosophie nehme,-- dargestellt an den Werken des Herrn Krug's,*" "*Verhältniss der Skepticismus zur Philosophie, Darstellung seiner verschiedenen Modificationen, und Vergleichung des neuesten mit dem alten,*" "*Glauben und Wissen oder ...,*" and "*Ueber die wissenschaftlichen Behandlungsarten des Naturrechts, seine Stelle in der praktischen Philosophie, und sein Verhältniss zu den positiven Rechtwissenschaften.*" It is generally accepted that the following pieces belong to Schelling: "*Ueber das absolute Identitäts-System und sein Verhältniss zu dem*

107

neuesten (Rheinholdischen) Dualismus," and *"Ueber Dante in philosophischer Beziehung."* The authorship of the remaining articles is still open to dispute. They are as follows: *"Rückert und Weiss, oder die Philosophie zu der es keines Denkens und Wissens bedarf," "Ueber das Verhältniss der Naturphilosophie zur Philosophie überhaupt,"* and *"Ueber die Construction in der Philosophie."*[3]

Aside from the question of authorship there is an involved matter concerning the originality of the individual pieces. Arguments have been marshalled both that Schelling was the more influential presence in the publication of the journal and that Hegel was.[4] Depending on which side one comes down upon, any given article could be read as a statement of the original philosophy of either author, no matter who did the writing. The circumstances under which the journal came to publication point in favor of taking Schelling as the leading thinker in the enterprise.[5] The history of thought, however, points in the other direction, as Hegel clearly emerged as the greater thinker of the two.

The idea of producing a leading journal of philosophy had been tossed about in Jena well before Hegel was on the scene. It is clear from correspondence of the period 1798-1802 that various influential figures considered participating in such a journal. Fichte, Schelling, Schleiermacher, and the Schlegel brothers all took part in an attempt to found a comprehensive critical journal. Squabbles broke out from the beginning between the players. By 1800 everyone had either been forced out or dropped out of his own accord, except Fichte and Schelling. Amidst promises that a journal would be forthcoming in 1801, the two remaining participants parted ways. Schelling, however, clung doggedly to the hope that such a journal could still be brought off. But it seems he would not proceed without a collaborator. When Hegel's first major publication, the *Differenz* essay, appeared in 1801, Schelling felt he had found his man.[6]

Late in 1800 Hegel had written a charming letter to Schelling, asking him to introduce him to the 'literary glut' in Jena. Schelling responded by inviting Hegel to co-produce the *Critical Journal of Philosophy.* Hegel responded with enthusiasm, suggesting straightaway that such a journal would be a fine forum for working out in detail some of the more interesting subjects introduced in the *Differenz* essay.[7]

Within a year of his overture to Schelling, Hegel was fairly champing at the bit, promising in a letter to W. F. Hufnagel, to use the new journal to "lay unphilosophical mischief low with cudgels, scourges and bats." The fiery spirit of this new critic is not diminished despite his son's later addition to the letter, claiming that the blows would be laid on in the name of the *gloriae Dei.*[8]

Though the idea of a critical journal of philosophy originally belonged to Schelling, Hegel quickly and most enthusiastically made it his own. And this in a manner that paved his way to fame as a great philosopher. For, as will become apparent in the analysis to follow, Hegel's contributions to the journal anticipate the form and content of his mature thought to the extent that, whatever their origin, they belong to his profoundly influential philosophy.

As it turns out, Hegel was clearly responsible for the bulk of the articles published in the journal. More importantly, the introductory article to the journal, which outlined the purpose of the journal and implicitly justified its content, was manifestly a product of Hegel's newfound role as a critic of the greatest philosophy Germany had to offer. For though this was a new vocation for Hegel, the current of critical thinking ran deep within him.[9]

A. The Idea of Criticism.

Hegel outlined the scope and aim of the new journal in the introductory article, "*Ueber das Wesen der philosophischen Kritik überhaupt, und ihr Verhältniss zum gegenwärtigen Zustand der Philosophie insbesondere*" (On the Essence of Philosophical Criticism in General and its Relation to the Present Condition of Philosophy in Particular). The guiding conception of criticism was: to identify and render clear the one and only idea of philosophy, as it was presented in the scientific systems of the day.[10]

The affinity with the notion of criticism set forth in the *Differenz* essay is clear: the idea of philosophy is rendered significant by setting it free within a system of thought. However, the dramatic lines in which Hegel previously portrayed the task of criticism are here drawn more starkly still. The image informing the present conception is of spirit rising out of the putrefaction of the deceased culture to a new life, soaring up from the ashes in rejuvenated form.[11]

To grasp what Hegel means by criticism here, we must explicate the connection between the idea of philosophy and the image of the phoenix. That connection, present in the wisdom of Plato and Montaigne, is expressed in the sceptical oracle that to philosophize is to learn to die.[12]

We begin with Hegel's model of criticism. The idea of philosophy, like that of art, is presupposed by and conditions philosophical criticism.[13] With the unchanging *Urbild der Sache selbst* at its origin, criticism applies a measure dependent neither upon the individual critic nor the work in question. Thus criticism can be objective in its judgments of art and philosophy only because the truth of reason, like beauty, is one.[14]

If, however, the idea of philosophy is not taken as the presupposition and condition of philosophical criticism, such criticism bears the mark of subjectivity. If the Absolute is conceived of as the mere object of philosophy, criticism can decide only on a subjective basis between a system which, for example, posits the Absolute as God and one which posits it as nature. Only by beginning with the unified idea of philosophy can criticism identify those systems which present the possibility of thinking the union of God and nature in the Absolute.[15]

Hegel outlines three forms in which the idea of philosophy can be discovered by the astute critic. The first is found in the 'beautiful soul':

> ... thus one must accept it with pleasure and gratification when the pure idea of philosophy expresses itself with spirit outside the scientific sphere as a naivete which does not attain to the objectivity of a systematic consciousness; it is the impression of a beautiful soul which had the inertness to preserve itself from the fall into thinking ...(SW Vol. 1, p. 176)[16]

The second form is apparent in a transitional stage of the 'beautiful soul', as portrayed in the remainder of the above passage:

> ... but it also lacked the courage to plunge itself into [the fall], and to work its guilt through to resolution; and for this reason it also did not attain in its self-intuition to an objective totality of science. (Ibid. p. 176f.)

The third and final form presents itself in the distinction emergent above between the desire for objectivity and objectivity itself:

> If it becomes clear here that the idea of philosophy is actually present to mind, criticism can adhere to the demand and to the desire which expresses itself, namely, the objective, wherein this desire seeks its satisfaction; and out of its proper, true tendency towards consummate objectivity, it can refute the limitation of its form. (Ibid. p. 177)[17]

Unless the unity of the Absolute presupposed by each of the forms above be taken as the ground of criticism, the critic must account for the possibility that there are various true philosophies. To attempt such an account, however, results in what Hegel calls the "spectacle of the torment of the damned," who are either eternally bound to their narrow-mindedness or admire in succession first this then that, casting one false truth away after another.[18]

Hegel thus distributes the sins of the damned under two basic types which represent the possibilities of failure both in philosophizing and in criticism. The first form of failure is met in systems of philosophy in which consciousness has not risen above subjectivity.[19]

The other possibility of failure presents itself in the form of technical philosophical terminology which only appears to harbor a genuine content within the obscurity of empty words.[20]

Though Hegel does not elaborate upon the interconnection of these two paths to failure, we might note the following. Because philosophy strives for objectivity, those systems in which consciousness remains subjective are especially prone to trade in technical terminology. For, by offering the terms of such systems as common currency in the marketplace of ideas, the subjectivity of consciousness assumes the shape of generality, and hence objectivity. But, as Hegel is so adamant to stress, the commonality of philosophical terminology is a false objectivity. It is merely the broad acceptance of a particular brand of subjectivity. And, even if such subjectivity were to become universal, still it would not be grounded in the only genuine form of objectivity, namely, the systematic presentation of the identity of subject and object in the Absolute.

When the propensity of subjective systems of thought for the false objectivity of terms held in common becomes explicit, it is clear that the critic's first concern is with the language of would-be philosophical systems. For, only by focusing primarily on terminology can the critic distinguish those systems of thought which conceal the kernel of the philosophic idea and those which comprise a mere whirl of terms without a kernel at their core. Thus the first task of the critic is to liberate the idea of philosophy from the many forms of philosophical jargon.[21]

Hegel's suggestion is the attempt to make a new beginning with philosophy and criticism. Lately philosophy had itself become 'critical', and so had taken over the task of criticism for itself.[22] The result was that both were the worse for the new arrangement. Philosophy had become critical of its idea, even to the point of denying that this idea could be known.[23] It had thereby swept the basis out from under itself and criticism. For how could one criticize philosophy, if philosophy itself lacked a defining idea? Hegel refused to see this as an advance. Far from being an innocent clearing of accounts in the name of further critical and philosophical ventures, this was the self-damning act of the leading minds of the day.

The rule of the day was that every philosopher worth his salt must work out the idea of philosophy according to his own individuality.[24] With this as the highest ideal of philosophy, lesser minds, and the public generally, were faced with the prospect of choosing from the host of individual systems.

So much was this the case that philosophy as such failed miserably. Rather than accepting the fate of being up-lifted by philosophy, the common person dragged philosophy down to the lowest level.[25] The people were led down a path marked by empty ideals and failed visions of humanity. A general unrest prevailed in which people strove in all directions after transient truths. The character of this fate was that of a dark feeling of mistrust and a secret doubt of philosophy.

The problem, according to Hegel, was that Cartesian philosophy had come to permeate modern culture, and its dualism marked the ruin of life.[26] The task laid upon the genuine critic of philosophy, then, was to liberate philosophy and thus the people for a thinking which superseded this dualism by returning to the identity of the Absolute:

> Every aspect of vital nature, and thus also philosophy, had to seek a means of escape from Cartesian philosophy and the general culture which expresses it. For Cartesianism has wrought in philosophical form the general, spreading dualism present in the culture of the recent history of our Northwestern world. The silent alteration of the public life of man, as also the loud political and religious revolutions are altogether only variegated superficies of this *dualism*, as of the decline of all old life. (Ibid. p. 187)

According to Hegel, the sole hope of philosophy rising from the ashes of Cartesianism[27] lay in modernity, and especially the German folk, submitting itself to the fate of the philosophic idea. For in this idea, and this idea alone, was to be found the unified source of life. It was the task of the *Critical Journal* to accomplish this destiny. Criticism, grounded upon the idea of philosophy, aimed at revealing the Absolute. If this could be adequately addressed and manifested through the criticism of philosophy, reason itself would likewise be presented in its totality, and with this the Absolute could be grasped in its infinity. By showing how various systems of philosophy embodied the kernel of the Absolute, criticism could identify the unity of philosophy. It was but one step further, albeit a very large one, to express the infinite in a system of philosophical (speculative) discourse.

Essential to Hegel's notion of philosophical criticism is his unique conception of reason. Most especially it is important to grasp how, according to Hegel, reason guides the criticism of philosophy. This matter warrants further attention.

That philosophy is one is apparent, according to Hegel, from the fact that reason is one. And reason, being one, cannot be separated from its self-knowledge. Thus no barrier can be posited between the reality of reason and the appearance of self-knowledge. Insofar as reason becomes an object for itself, it is philosophy, and as reason, philosophy is one. Thus the nemesis of philosophical criticism is the infinity of various reflections upon reason as an object for but not of consciousness. For in all such reflections there exists a rift between the subject and its object. And, whether reason be objectified as God or as nature, reflective philosophy splits the subject from that which it desires to know. To this extent such philosophy is unphilosophical. Philosophy, properly so called, must rest upon the unity of the self-consciousness of the Absolute. Philosophical criticism, then, is possible only where the idea of philosophy is present in its oneness. To this extent, criticism presupposes speculation, both as the pre-reflective grasp of the Absolute and as its post-reflective expression in thought.

By Hegel's own account philosophical criticism was impossible at the time when he undertook to present its concept to the public. Yet this was not because the presupposition of speculation was misplaced. Much rather criticism had lost the idea of philosophy amidst the practice of shouting others down in favor of the latest and most authoritative subjectivism. More than this, philosophy itself had lost its idea, for it lamely took its lead from the then current spirit of criticism. But Hegel's insight was that in the impossibility of genuine criticism was to be found a contradiction, and from out of this contradiction itself could arise the renewed possibility of both criticism and philosophy.

The contradiction in question was that subjective criticism attempted to become objective through asserting itself as subjectively more persuasive and forceful than any other criticism. Consent to a subjective point of view here counted as objectivity, when such consent was deemed common or universal. But such criticism is only an intensification of subjectivism, for no criticism can become objective by throwing away the oneness of philosophy. The oneness of philosophy is not one by common consent, but by virtue of the nature of philosophy itself. Thus subjective criticism not only lacks objectivity, it is in fact through and through a negative affair. Ever and again casting away the idea of philosophy, subjective criticism is unphilosophical. It has a merely negative relation to philosophy, and can never be transformed into something positive. The course taken by such criticism, generally considered, then, is the serial of nothing, the unfolding of an infinite nihilism.

By bringing subjective criticism low, Hegel clears a way for his more positive, objective conception of criticism. He proposes that now attention must be paid to those systems of philosophy which incorporate the idea of philosophy in its unity. The critic has merely to tease that idea out of the system, render it clear, and comprehend its significance. However, as mentioned above, the philosophy of the day had itself lost the idea, having taken its lead from subjectivist criticism. Thus Hegel's task must be taken as twofold: to destroy subjective criticism, and to replace philosophy to a position superior to that of criticism as such. The problem of course was to do this from the subordinate station of a critic.

In keeping with this task, Hegel proffers here no new philosophy. This would be to commit the error of the past philosophers. Instead he employs his lower position as a critic to conjure the lofty philosophical idea in systems which are in fact lacking with respect to that idea. In short, he makes use of a hermeneutical prerogative of the critic: to see more in a work than does the author.

Initially Hegel points to the idea of philosophy in the expressions of a beautiful soul, that soul which withholds itself from the fall into thinking, even as it thinks. For, even if it is apparent that this soul lacks the courage to work through its 'guilt' toward resolution in a properly philosophical system, still it portrays in an instant a certain naivete of spirit.[29] And that naivete is the kernel of philosophy.

The critic can cause the seed of philosophy to germinate and grow forth, if the two aforementioned sorts of failure can be avoided. First, the consciousness of the critic must not remain subjective, but must instead develop to the point at which it can be shown that the work in question is the form of the idea. Second, the critic must not render the form of the idea in empty words and phrases borrowed from the common market of unphilosophical platitudes. The critic must instead employ living forms of language. This amounts to enlivening the idea by liberating it from the strictures of what Hegel calls the critical philosophy, or the philosophy of reflection.

Hegel cites Kant's philosophy as an example of a system that possesses the kernel of the philosophic idea. This philosophy presents reason in its self-recognition. Here there is a glimpse of reason considering itself as an object:

> In this respect the critical philosophy performed an excellent service. Namely, in that it has demonstrated (in order to render it in the terminology of that philosophy) that the concepts of the understanding have their application only in experience; that reason knowingly entangled itself in contradictions through its theoretical ideas; and that knowledge generally must be given its objects through sensibility. (Ibid. p. 181)

However, because the form of such self-recognition is contradiction (it appears in the form of antinomies), the criticism and development of Kantian philosophy by others has led to a dismissal of reason as such, and a consequent entrenchment in the crassest empiricism.

Kant's philosophy, because it presents itself as absolute without regard for the difficulty of portraying subjectivity as a system, becomes the bad conscience of philosophical criticism. And, it would seem, the negative depiction of reason in Kant's philosophy provides criticism with a *carte blanche* for its bad conscience. Reason is so degraded that it is conceived merely as an hypothesis for theoretical constructs or as a postulate of practical affairs. Hence it can in no way function as the guide for philosophical criticism.

Once philosophy has thus squandered its idea in a distorted conception of reason, it becomes the task of saving the finite. The finite is equated with the true, and the Absolute becomes an inaccessible beyond. To assuage the bad conscience of criticism, philosophy sets about to present certainty as its necessary starting point. The notion of a pure self-consciousness is advanced, and is supposed to be set over against the empirical. In actuality, however, pure self-consciousness is nothing more than the mere limit of the empirical, and so belongs to the empirical. Such a philosophy tries to tie itself fast to certainties by drawing upon facts recognized by human understanding as belonging to the common good. But either this is superfluous to philosophy proper, which by its nature must surpass common sense, or it is to present the infinite as that toward which finitude should tend, but which can never be attained. The criticism informing such philosophy strives to popularize, or render common, these propositions and constructs, and in so doing becomes a hindrance both to philosophy and to common understanding. It is manifestly not the case that a bad conscience becomes the better by being held in common.

Philosophy, according to Hegel, is esoteric by nature. It is not fashioned for the masses, nor can it be made palatable to the masses. Philosophy is philosophical to the extent that it is set against the local and temporary limitations of a given culture. The obvious example here is Socrates, who philosophized against the people of Athens even unto death. In relation to the common world, the world of philosophy is an inverted, topsy-turvy world. Yet it is the task of philosophy to raise the people for this world, without itself stooping into their world.

In Hegel's opinion, the above idea of philosophy was the only hope to be held out for his native culture. To be sure, it was no ripe fruit, hanging heavy on the tree of knowledge, within easy grasp. It was, as Hegel mentions several times, much less even than this: it was a mere kernel, hidden under several husks. But the critic, by peeling each husk away increasingly brought the possibility of such an idea nearer fruition.

But perhaps even this is too much to say. For the kernel mentioned in the body of the essay is eclipsed at the end by the image of the phoenix. An image more powerful than an agrarian myth was required for Hegel to make his difficult point. The phoenix metaphor depicted the gravity of criticism. The boredom of philosophy would have to be stirred up into a yearning for riches--with a drop of fire, a concentration of living intuition, and, after death has been known long enough, with an appreciation of the living.

This would be possible only through reason. The critic could only be effective by aspiring to the idea of philosophy, by taking upon himself the fate of reason. To mix the metaphors of the fruit and the phoenix, the hulls could not be stripped away from the kernel, save that the critic be consumed by the philosophical drop of fire. The critic would have to suffer the fall of the beautiful soul into thinking, before he could rise from the ashes and enjoy the fruition of the idea of philosophy.[30] To criticize, for Hegel, would be to die the death of a philosopher.

B. Common Sense

In this section we will consider Hegel's first article in the *Critical Journal*. But, before attention can be turned upon this, further comments are in order regarding the form and content of the journal.

The *Critical Journal* taken as a whole represents a loosely constructed program for the cure of the philosophical boredom which lay at the heart of modern culture. Hegel himself, however, does not refer to the journal articles as comprising such a program, except in the broad sense outlined in the introductory article.[31] He merely develops the idea of philosophical criticism, and the reader must pick up the flow in the articles themselves. A cursory examination of the contents of the journal attributed to him, however, makes the outlines of the implicit program clear.

The first article of Hegel's to appear in the journal, *Wie der gemeine Menschenverstand die Philosophie nehme, -dargestellt an den Werken des Herrn Krug's* (How Common Human Understanding Would Take Philosophy; Portrayed through the Works of Krug), considers a system of philosophy that represents the simplest and most naive kind of knowledge to go under the name of philosophy, i.e., empiricism. Hegel had identified empiricism in the introduction to the journal as the product of the critical philosophy of Kant.[32] Immediately following this is an article on scepticism entitled *Verhältniss des Skepticismus zur Philosophie, Darstellung seiner verschiedenen Modificationen, und Vergleichung des neuesten mit dem alten* (The Relation of Scepticism to Philosophy, a Portrayal of its Different Modifications, and a Comparison of the Latest Scepticism to Ancient Scepticism). This article represents the next level of knowledge in philosophical writings. Here is a philosophy, called scepticism, that accepts the certainties of empiricism, but rejects all constructive claims made by reason. Next in Hegel's repertoire is the article on faith and knowledge, which scrutinizes the philosophy of reflection represented by the systems of Kant, Jacobi, and Fichte. This philosophy is presented as the most sophisticated statement of knowledge to date, as it touches upon the role of reason as both regulative and as constructive.[33] The last of Hegel's articles in the journal is the essay on natural law, dealing with the scientific treatment of the concept of right. This article outlines a yet more complex and sophisticated role for reason in philosophy, focusing upon the crucial question of thinking aright and acting properly.

Thus if the pieces attributable to Hegel are considered in isolation from the rest of the material, it becomes apparent that his contribution to the journal, not only provides a program for the cure of philosophical and cultural malaise, but also represents the development of consciousness from sense-certainty to absolute knowledge which appears some years later in the *Phenomenology of Spirit*.[34]

In the first article of the journal, on "How common human understanding would take philosophy," Hegel sets his idea of philosophical criticism to work upon a then major figure. Wilhelm Traugott Krug (1770-1842) occupied a chair in philosophy at Frankfurt on the Oder at the time Hegel's review article came out, and two years later he was to become Kant's successor at Königsberg.[35]

As we shall see, Krug had presented a systematic philosophy in eight volumes that was to rectify the problems which had lately arisen in the transcendental idealism of Fichte and Schelling. The task was to replace the complex and difficult notion of an absolute ego, crucial in the systems of both idealists, with a streamlined version of empirical consciousness.

Krug's philosophy was a good target for Hegel's criticism because it promised a system of knowledge, and did so by veering away from reason. On the surface, then, Krug appeared to hold out hope for Hegel's idea of a unified, systematic philosophy, but on a deeper level he seemed to undermine the connection between that idea and reason. If Krug was correct, manifestly Hegel was wrong in proposing that reason was the medium of systematic philosophy. Hegel thus put his idea of philosophy to the test by gauging it in relation to the last great philosophical system of the day.

In analyzing Hegel's review article, I will present first his description of Krug's philosophical system, second his negative criticisms of the individual claims which make up that system, and third his comprehended suggestions as to the truth of the matter at hand. This division of Hegel's comments into three distinct elements is admittedly artificial. In the course of the article itself Hegel runs all three together in massive, tortuous sentences. However, there is in these passages often a discernible pattern of positing, negating, and comprehending. The following excerpts, translated in sequence from a long paragraph make the point clear:

> ... [Krug] requires only a little something, only the deduction of a particular representation, for example, the moon with all of its features .... But does Mr. Krug have so little a conception of philosophical construction to suggest that the moon could be comprehended without

the entire solar system? And does he have so weak a representation of this solar system that he fails to see that the knowing of this system is the most sublime and highest task of reason?

We see here how the deduction of a particular representation is negated by the imposition of a representation of totality, which then is presented as a cure for the weakened grasp of reason betrayed in the desire for such a deduction.

I will not present each of the major points of the article in the above fashion, but will segregate them according to their type. In this way we will have a heightened sense of the unity and totality of Hegel's emergent idea of philosophy as represented in his comprehensive comments on common sense.

Hegel describes Krug's position as having two basic elements. The first is its polemic against the *Wissenschaftslehre* of Fichte and the new idealism of Schelling. The second is its presentation of certain philosophic convictions which Krug himself had developed.

As regards the former element, Krug took transcendental idealism to task over its conception of the ego. Transcendental idealism had taken the proper first step in putting the ego forth as the basis of a philosophical system, but had gone astray in conceiving of this ego as an absolute subject, ultimately divorced from all experiential reality.

Hegel thus notes that Krug takes transcendental idealism seriously, even to the point of accepting its initial step: "Take notice of yourself, avert your gaze from everything that surrounds you, and turn it inward."[36]

The inner-self of reflective thinking is, in Krug's judgment, the ground for all philosophy. But transcendental idealism mistakes this ground by dogmatically asserting that the ego defines its own limits, not through freedom and arbitrariness, but according to an immanent law belonging to its eternal essence. Such a notion of the ego is informed by the philosophical interest in discovering a self-standing subject. But, Krug counters, as regards this interest itself, it is of no concern whether the ego is limited by external factors or by its nature: the music of a harp, for instance, is no different whether it is played by a musician or the wind, except that the former is more obviously musical than the latter. Transcendental idealism, then, complicates matters by maintaining that philosophical knowledge arises from the inner nature of the ego, rather than from the effect of the external world upon the ego. The consequence of this complication is that the reality of the external world is called into question. It is at this point, according to Hegel, that Krug takes leave of the idealist philosophy.[37]

A related polemic against transcendental idealism concerns the matter of morality, or practical reason. Apparently because transcendental idealism posits a self-standing subject determined by its innermost laws, it is ultimately indifferent toward matters of duty and the like. As Krug would have it, the idealist would fail to save a drowning person, because he/she would hesitate too long, frozen in the face of the incomprehensibility of the obstacles involved. It seems Krug has in mind that whatever does not arise from the inner nature of the ego (e.g., the obstacles involved in saving the drowning person) will confound the transcendental idealist, because such matters defy a deduction from the ego.

A third criticism Krug levels against the philosophy of Fichte and Schelling is that, though transcendental idealism is to be a philosophy without presupposition, it presupposes the very basis of the ego itself, namely, the absolute A=A.[38]

Krug's final opposition to transcendental idealism arises over the claim that the total system of our representations can be deduced from the absolute ego. So little is transcendental idealism capable of providing this deduction, Krug maintains, that it cannot even deduce a single determinate object. But if Fichte and Schelling cannot deduce even Krug's feather pen, how can they deduce the totality of all representations?[39]

In addition to his criticisms of transcendental idealism Krug presents certain philosophical convictions in his work. Hegel lists these convictions as follows. First, there is in our consciousness a primordial transcendental synthesis between the real and the ideal. This inexplicable truth forms the basis of a system Krug calls Synthecism.[40] Second, the ego is the reality of the transcendental synthesis. That the ego is indeed real follows from the reality of states of consciousness generally and acts of consciousness in particular. Not even the sceptic can deny that behind all real actions lies a real subject.[41] Third, consciousness is contained within the ego, and is a collection of an infinite variety of things, e.g., the principle of non-contradiction, duty, Alexander the Great, etc. As such consciousness is a wholly unordered chaos. Hegel puts it as follows:

> To be sure, these infinitely manifold facts of consciousness all lie in the I, into which they all come in an incomprehensible manner, but indeed like chaos, without any unity or order:
>> Everything is mixed, one through another
>> like mouse crap and coriander. (Ibid. p. 206)

Fourth, reason provides a formal unity to the chaos of consciousness. Each fact of consciousness is known by the subject as its own. This collection of facts is, according to Krug, reason itself.[42] Fifth, there is one principle of reality, namely, the ego, and several principles of ideality, e.g., the external world, God, etc.[43]

In sum, Krug's philosophical convictions comprise a system of an infinite chain of limitations in empirical consciousness. One state of consciousness is cancelled in the flow of empirical perception, then preserved in the infinity of consciousness, and then the next state of consciousness is already upon the subject. The movement of cancelling and preserving the facts of consciousness is, according to Krug, the organon of philosophy. Hegel, however, describes this organon as a mere composite of popular philosophical opinions:

> According to the prevailing [philosophy] the synthecism of Mr. Kr. must be thought in the following way: one imagines for oneself a pitcher, wherein Reinholdian water, flat Kantian beer, enlightening syrup called Berlinism, and other like ingredients are contained as facts by means of some sort of coincidence. But now a person steps up, and thereby brings a unity into the mess, so that he separates the things, sniffs and tastes one after the other, or as it is done, hears mainly from others what has found its way in [the mix], and then renders an account of this. Now this is formal unity, or philosophical consciousness. (Ibid. p. 208)

Built into Hegel's presentation of Krug's philosophy is his criticism, both positive and negative. First the negative side. Hegel takes up various points expressed by Krug to illumine the mistaken way in which Krug has taken hold of the basic elements of German philosophy. Krug, Hegel asserts, has simply misunderstood the philosophy of transcendental idealism, and so his criticisms of Fichte and Schelling miss the mark. Moreover, Krug's embracing of the ego as the basic principle of reality does a disservice to the idealist philosophy. Hegel maintains against Krug that the philosophy of transcendental idealism does not call into question the existence of the external world, and so actually stands in no need of Krug's supposed deduction of that world from the reality of the ego. The idealist philosophy, Hegel avers, affirms both the reality and the ideality of the external world. Moreover, the theoretical portion of the *Wissenschaftslehre* of Fichte is concerned with nothing but a deduction of the reality of the external world.[44]

Next Hegel takes Krug to task over the apparent grand contradiction at the heart of transcendental idealism, namely, that it presupposes the identity and difference of the ego (the absolute principle, A=A), even though it professes to be a philosophy without presupposition. This contradiction, Hegel states, is precisely that which common understanding always finds in philosophy: common understanding places the Absolute on the same rung as the finite, and applies to the Absolute the same claims as are properly made only with respect to the finite, e.g., that nothing in philosophy can be admitted without proof, even and especially the Absolute. Krug's claim is that transcendental idealism has failed to prove the existence of the Absolute. Hegel counters that the Absolute is in no need of such proof, for it is not just one contingent thing among others. Proper attention to reason would make as much clear, but common sense insists upon the findings of the understanding: just because we can form an idea of something does not mean that the thing necessarily exists.[45]

Hegel remarks that if Krug is consistent in applying the notion of a presuppositionless system of thought, he will be forced to cast geometry aside, for it does not prove the existence of the infinite space in which it draws its lines. Does Krug wish to argue that philosophy is guilty of holding God or the Absolute as a hypothesis, just as one physics postulates empty space and another magnetic matter?[46]

Hegel next draws attention to Krug's claim that philosophy is grounded in consciousness. Hegel's position is that the transcendental synthesis of states of consciousness cannot serve as the foundation for a philosophy, for consciousness is not basic. Though Krug maintains that the primordial synthesis is consciousness, Hegel reminds that consciousness is still but a part of the ego. The ego, then, and not mere consciousness must provide the ground for philosophy.[47]

Krug is again criticized over his treatment of the ego, but this time it is in a more obvious connection with the question of reason. Krug wanted to follow the lead of transcendental idealism in placing the ego as the basis of a system of knowing. But because he insisted, against transcendental idealism, that the ego is consciousness as such, he undermined the relation of the ego to reason, a connection essential to the philosophy of idealism. Hegel points out that Krug merely employs reason as a term by which to explain more fully what he has in mind by consciousness.[48]

Reason is not considered in its own right in the whole of the eight volumes of Krug's work reviewed by Hegel. This, Hegel notes, is precisely because reason cannot be made into a thing in the way that the ego as consciousness is a simple thing.

Hegel again returns to the question of reason, criticizing Krug for bringing reason into the picture merely as a formal unity for the states of consciousness. Reason is that ordering and ranking of the whirling chaos of the facts of consciousness. Hegel compares reason in this capacity to the coping-stone of an arch that draws attention to itself as the highest and last stone of the structure. The unity of the stones is thus present in the completion of the structure. But, though the highest and the last of stones, the coping-stone does not include in itself the foundation of the arch.[49] The unity it provides the manifold of stones, then, falls far short of an all-encompassing, grounding unity. Thus in Krug's system reason is, as Hegel puts it, brought in in the genetive. No real attempt is made to show that reason is anything more than merely the last piece to fall into place in Krug's philosophical edifice.

Hegel's final point against Krug also has to do with reason. Krug expresses his aspiration to present an organon for philosophy, but as it turns out this is not provided in his eight volumes. Hegel concedes that Krug has at any rate provided a charming seven-volume collection of the facts of consciousness. Still he wonders (sarcastically) that the number of volumes was perhaps too few to include the infinitely manifold facts of philosophical consciousness. Hegel then concludes his article on common sense by remarking that, even if seven volumes were enough to contain consciousness, where is there supposed to be any room for philosophizing over these matters that have been laid down as the ground of knowledge, since the eighth and final volume is taken up by bibliographical materials and an index of the things included in the previous seven volumes?[50]

In sum, Hegel's negative criticisms of Krug center on the issue of reason in philosophy. Common human understanding takes up with philosophy by attaching itself to an empirical positivism which suppresses or otherwise excludes the role of reason in human knowledge. But, if this step is taken, one has already set out upon a path leading away from true philosophy. To forfeit the matter of reason is to acquiesce to a conception of philosophy which is less than consummately unified. Reason alone provides a route to the idea of philosophy embraced by Hegel in his critical writing, for only it can encompass the reality of philosophical half-truths or outright errors. Only reason can fashion the shortcomings of opinion into the totality of truth. A view to the positive side of Hegel's review will show how he recognizes Krug's errors, rejects them, and finally comprehends them in portraying a constructive, burgeoning idea of philosophy.

The first important constructive remark Hegel makes in the article is that the being of the Absolute is immediately posited in its idea. The remark is made in response to Krug's claim that transcendental idealism presupposes the absolute A=A as absolute identity and difference. Thus the comment conveys that the Absolute is not in need of the sorts of proofs required for finite things. However, common understanding refuses to recognize this, claiming that it can very well think of something without at the same time positing its existence. But the Absolute, according to Hegel, is neither one thing alongside other things in need of proof nor one hypothesis alongside of other hypotheses proffered by any given system of knowledge. Much rather the Absolute is that which in being thought is.[51]

Hegel's second constructive remark expands upon the first. Philosophy, he notes, has been long enough concerned with God as one finitude among others or as a postulate for an absolute finitude. The immediate task of philosophy, Hegel presses, is to replace God to the summit of philosophy as the sole ground of the All, as the single *principium essendi* and *cognoscendi.*[52] In criticizing Krug's challenge that the transcendental philosophy deduce the reality of even a single thing, Hegel alludes to this loftier notion of philosophy, based in the unity of being and knowing, the real and the ideal: the Absolute.

Third, Hegel responds enthusiastically to Krug's assertion that philosophy must have at its starting point a unity of the real and the ideal. Krug, again, maintained that there was in consciousness an original synthesis of the real and the ideal, which makes possible an inseparable connection between transcendental realism and transcendental idealism. These words, Hegel remarks, sound good indeed. All of them, that is, save the term, synthesis. This word, Hegel warns, does not do justice to the matter. And it is Krug's reliance upon the notion of a synthesis that leads him to place consciousness before the ego in his philosophy, and consequently to make the mistake of divorcing the ego from reason. For, apparently, if the ego had been placed first, the connection between it and reason would have become manifest. Hegel's way of dealing with the matter, then, suggests that reason is to be proffered as a constructive, and not merely regulative, term in the matter of philosophy.

Finally, Hegel refers to the notion of a genuine philosophical system as one which encompasses in itself all others at once. The comment is made in the context of a negative criticism against Krug's system: it is not easy to see how the essence of the Krugian synthesis makes room for an all-encompassing philosophical system, because it in fact does not.[53] As the remark about whether Krug's eight volumes · are enough to encompass philosophy makes clear, Hegel's notion of a genuine philosophical system is not merely the quantitative idea of the entire contents of philosophy. This matter of quantity does seem to play some part, in as much as the history of philosophy is crucial to philosophizing (a point which will become abundantly clear in the section to follow, on Hegel's next critical review). But here the emphasis is rather on finding the content of philosophy that will raise philosophizing to a higher form. The remarks about the task of comprehending the solar system in its totality, and that of recognizing God as the unity of being and knowing are to be taken in this sense. Or, to return to the example of the stone arch, the true philosophical system will be such that its coping-stone is at once the foundation of the edifice itself.

That this is a difficult thought goes without saying. And that Hegel does not make it any easier in his review article is also obvious to the reader. The piecemeal allusions to such a system of philosophy do more to point back to the concept of criticism presented in the journal's introductory article than forward to any presentation of the truly comprehensive philosophy.[54] So much is this the case that reason, so important to the system to come, comes into play in the review of Krug's work only in a critical role. Reason is held out as that which Krug's philosophy fails to address, and even suppresses. But to the extent that Hegel's article is materially bound to Krug's philosophy, reason cannot come up of its own. The entire article spins a fine web that ultimately entangles Krug in the trap of common human understanding. And by implication, Kant too is made out to be a philosopher of the understanding. Hegel too is bound to common understanding and the fact of consciousness, but the tie that binds him is speculative criticism. This is the measure of his freedom. For, even while having nothing more than a negative conception of the understanding, Hegel is compelled toward something which lies beyond common philosophy. The idea of a necessary being, the Absolute or God, the totality of the solar system, the unwritten organon of Krug's philosophy, all conspire toward that beyond. The gap between Krug's philosophy and the philosophy of transcendental idealism is in fact the problematic of consciousness and reason exposed by criticism. But the vastness of this gap requires that a systematic approach be taken in order to construct a bridge from the fragmentary facts of consciousness to the speculative totality of reason.

The next article to be taken in sequence (on scepticism and philosophy) will heighten the sense of Hegel's anticipation of the true philosophy. In his critical rehearsal of the history of thought Hegel will establish the basis for the freedom to think.

C. Scepticism.

The next article to appear in the journal bears the title, *Verhältniss des Skepticismus zur Philosophie; Darstellung seiner verschiedenen Modifikationen, und Vergleichung des neuesten mit dem alten* (The Relation of Scepticism to Philosophy, a Portrayal of its Different Modifications, and a Comparison of the Latest Scepticism to Ancient Scepticism).[55] Here Hegel sets out to demonstrate a necessary connection between the one true form of philosophy, as mentioned in the introduction to the journal, and all types of scepticism. In so doing he takes up with the latest presentation of scepticism, in Gottlob Ernst Schulze's *Kritik der theoretischen Philosophie* (Bohn: 1801). Hegel exposes the origin of this latter-day scepticism to lie in the genuine scepticism of the ancients. He then portrays scepticism as such as the negative side of the speculative philosophy of the Absolute.

This article thus serves to further develop Hegel's emergent idea of philosophy by rendering all forms of scepticism as greater or lesser representations of an aspect or moment of that philosophy.[56] What had appeared in the journal's introductory article as the negative work of criticism now emerges under the name of scepticism, as the negative side of the one true philosophy.

The important step here is that what the critic merely found lacking in the presentation of a philosophical system such as Krug's is now posited as the presupposition of all negative approaches to such systems. If reason is what was lacking in Krug's philosophy, scepticism is what enabled Hegel to divine this. Scepticism lurks within all such positive systems of common sense. Indeed it represents the freedom of the system itself to reflect upon and even challenge its most basic concepts from within. But without the positive presentation of the system as the appearance of reason under the guise of common sense, scepticism itself withers away.

In one simple move Hegel's idea of an all-encompassing philosophy is doubled in size and strength, by including within itself all forms that oppose it.

Hegel describes Schulze's aim as the destruction of theoretical philosophy through a new scepticism. Hegel essays to gauge the true worth of this scepticism, first by measuring it in relation to ancient scepticism, and then by comparing it with philosophy proper. Thereby Hegel attempts to determine when it is more reasonable to doubt than to be certain.[57]

Hegel examines Schulze's depiction of the source of his scepticism. The new scepticism contains the discourse of thoughts that supposedly arises from a knowing based in reason, but which fails to win universal approval for itself.[58] The participants of this discourse stand in a deadlock of contradictions. Every new attempt to give the knowledge in question the substance of science miscarries. Thus it becomes clear that the goal of this knowledge is unattainable, and that all of the participants share a common error.[59]

Schulze's description is of the malaise of German philosophy that had settled in, in the wake of Kant's great work on theoretical reason. No one had been able to capitalize on Kant's problematic theory of knowledge. The wide-ranging disputes about what Kant had really meant testified to this. Indeed it seemed, that for all the initial enthusiasm, the Kantian theoretical philosophy ultimately promised nothing but the failure to philosophize. And what held for Kant's theory of knowledge held as well for all theoretical philosophy.

Hegel retorts that this is a very subjective way of putting the matter. Schulze, Hegel charges, has lost his nerve for theoretical philosophy because he has seen the failure of such great figures as Kant and his followers.

This loss of confidence on Schulze's part is, according to Hegel, the suppression of the capacity to philosophize. It is to become fixated upon the fate met by all speculative pursuits grounded in our knowledge of the existence of things.[60] To be so fixated, however, is to give oneself and philosophy over to an ill fate. Hegel compares Schulze's way of putting the matter of philosophy to the predicament of a political protester in ancient Greece:

> At the time when unrest broke out in the city, the Athenian lawgivers set [the penalty of] death for political *apragmosyne*. Philosophical *apragmosyne* --not to espouse a party, but to be decided in advance to submit oneself to that fate which would be crowned with victory and universality-- is of itself cursed with the death of speculative reason. (SW Vol. 1, p. 217)

Just as the Athenian love of political ease sealed the fate of Socrates, so Schulze's love of philosophical ease -his desire to ground philosophy in the general consent to propositions- entails the death of speculative philosophy.[61]

Hegel's analogy poses the unrest of the people, stirred by philosophy, and speculative reason on one side, and the sentence of death and the new scepticism on the other side. Thus the love of ease in matters political and philosophical ultimately leads to both the death of the people and of speculative reason.[62]

Such a relation between philosophy and politics would dictate that what is most properly philosophical is that which resists common sense.[63] Hence, in order to find what is genuinely philosophical in a common philosophy, it is necessary to critically search out the uncommon in it. But, because the new scepticism focuses exclusively upon the failure of philosophy to become common, it fails to consider this fate itself as a moment of philosophy; it equates the fate of the uncommon with the end of philosophy itself. Schulze thus places difference (dispute) before unity (unanimity) in philosophy. But Hegel retorts that difference, division, conflict in philosophy presupposes unity:

> But the old rule: *contra negantes principia non est disputandum* indicates already that when philosophical systems struggle with one another unity of the principles is present, which is superior to every success or fate. (Ibid. p. 218)

Schulze, however, concludes from the fact of a philosophical struggle that what the combatants share is an error. This error, according to Schulze, lies in the very power of human knowing, and so we cannot look to the future for success in speculative philosophy.[64]

Hegel, for his part, has nothing more to say about this alleged error. But the definition of theoretical philosophy attributed to Schulze by Hegel seems to imply what that error would be. Schulze distinguishes theoretical from practical and aesthetic philosophy, and dismisses the latter two. Theoretical philosophy he considers to be the following: the science of the highest and unconditioned causes of all conditioned things, but of whose reality we are uncertain.[65]

The error referred to is apparently that speculative reason claims to know the unconditioned causes of all that is, despite the fact, or so Schulze would have it, that to know something is for it to be conditioned. Thus, Schulze maintains, speculation, as the act of knowing unconditioned causes, is self-contradictory, and so can be nothing but an error. Unconditioned causes, he avers, are like rocks beneath the snow: they lie back of the objects of perception received in natural consciousness. These causes, he concludes, are discovered in their hidden reality solely through the use of concepts and principles, and not through direct knowledge or immediate intuition.[66]

Hegel's consideration of Schulze's scepticism is designed in part to dispel the notion that philosophical disputes arise from the 'error' of speculation. To this end he presents Schulze's scepticism in two parts. The first, what Hegel calls the positive side of the scepticism, comprises Schulze's theory of consciousness.

Schulze promises a philosophy that does not overstep the bounds of consciousness, and yet one that maintains the indubitable certainty of the existence of those things given in consciousness. According to Schulze, we can no more doubt those things given in consciousness than we can doubt consciousness itself. It is, he proposes, absolutely impossible to doubt consciousness, because to do so presupposes the consciousness necessary to doubt. What is given in consciousness are the facts of consciousness, the indubitably real, to which all philosophical speculation must bind itself, and which is explained and made comprehensible through speculation.[67]

The positive aspect of Schulze's scepticism, then, is that consciousness mediates all knowledge. As such it stands between speculation and its intended object. Thus the facts of empirical consciousness are placed before the claims of speculative reason, and so serve to regulate those claims.[68]

Hegel's presentation of the so-called negative side of Schulze's scepticism is somewhat more involved. Here Hegel considers what scepticism as such is.

According to Schulze, the difference between his new scepticism and that of the ancients lies in what each doubts. Ancient scepticism, in Schulze's account, doubted the teachings of experience. This entailed questioning or even rejecting the content of external sensations. It also involved the dismissal of the sciences, as these were based upon experience.[69] The new scepticism, however, doubts only the science of philosophy, and this only to the extent that it attempts to go beyond the bounds of consciousness.[70]

The origin and development of ancient scepticism was determined, according to Schulze, in relation to the presumptions of dogmatic philosophy. The ancients accepted that there is a knowing through the senses, and even a conviction arising from the senses of the existence and given characteristics of abiding things. It was according to this knowledge that every reasonable person was thought to direct the practical affairs of life. But just because such knowing had only to do with practical life, Schulze deduces, it is clear that such scepticism had nothing to do with philosophy itself. The ancient sceptic did not even attempt to raise this consciousness of things to the level of scientific knowledge. Sextus Empiricus, says Schulze, maintained that the sceptic attended to the appearances of consciousness only to the extent that was necessitated by the affairs of practical living.[71]

It is regarding this last point that Hegel presents his substantive criticisms of Schulze's account of scepticism. Hegel responds that the ancient sceptic made no claim to a conviction about the existence and characteristics of things, not even for matters of practice. Much rather the ancient sceptic focused upon that which appears (*phainomenon*), claiming that it was mere appearance (*phantasian autou*) and the subjective.[72] But, Hegel reminds, the ancient sceptic meant by 'the subjective' that which is unexamined (*azetetos*).[73]

And so the ancient sceptic doubted perception to the extent that it involved unexamined appearance:

> But the sceptics account for all perception as mere semblance, instead of subscribing to its indisputable certainty, and they affirm that one would just as well have to assert the opposite of that which one would have said about the object with respect to its appearance -- to say just as well that honey is bitter, as [that it is] sweet ... (Ibid. p. 227)

The issue was, according to Hegel, the examination of both sides of appearance.

Thus, Hegel argues, more important than the doubting of the claims of dogmatic philosophy (e.g., that there is a rock beneath the snow) in favor of perceptions which serve common sense was the critical examination of perception as such:

> When the sceptic said: Honey is just as bitter as sweet, and just as sweet as bitter, there was no intended thing posited behind honey. (Ibid. p. 227f.)

From this consideration of the claims of ancient scepticism Hegel concludes that, if Schulze's thinking is to properly bear the name of scepticism, it must relinquish its common sense claim to the certainty of perceptions. Furthermore, it must be seen that the true origin of this latter-day, so-called scepticism lies, not in some alleged ancient scepticism which set itself against dogmatic philosophy, but rather in the innermost truth of scepticism as such. This genuine scepticism, Hegel avers, is one with every true philosophy, a philosophy which is neither sceptical nor dogmatic, in the limited sense of these terms.[74]

Hegel develops this notion of scepticism through a comment of Diogenes Laertius:

> However, Diogenes Laertius himself advances in his way that some name Homer as the founder of scepticism, because he speaks differently of the same things in different situations; so also many of the sayings of the Seven Sages are sceptical ... but Diogenes further cites Archikochus, Euripides, Zeno, Xenophanes, Democritus, Plato, etc., as sceptics ... (Ibid. p. 230)

Hegel's interpretation is that each of the persons mentioned shared in the insight that a true philosophy also necessarily has a negative side which turns against all limitation, and so against the confines of the facts of consciousness and its alleged indubitable certainty.

Hegel characterizes this root sense of scepticism according to the philosophy of Plato. With regard to Plato scepticism directs itself not against reason, but against that claim to knowledge which bases itself upon the world of appearance.[75] Plato's philosophy is a total negation of the truth and reality of knowledge that sees things as manifold pieces divided from out of the whole construed in a process of arising and passing away.

With regard to the others the point is more difficult to grasp. Homer and Euripides, for instance, do not seem to share Plato's philosophical aversion to the transitory. Hegel says nothing in particular about these so-called sceptics, but one might venture that the scepticism of Plato expressed with respect to the transitory things of sensation and consciousness is reflected in the Homeric art of portraying the same thing differently in differing circumstances. For, though Plato spoke out against such an art in his *Republic*, still he would perhaps recognize a genuine truth in Homer's refusal to adhere to any given appearance of empirical reality.[76] Thus Homer's crafted perspectivalism, as it were, is a faithful representation of the transitory nature of empirical consciousness. This in itself is in keeping with the Platonic philosophy.

By fashioning various representations of the phenomena of perception, Homer indicates that his art is not committed to the absoluteness of any given form of appearance. Apparently it is because of just some such insight into the scepticism of the ancients that Hegel is able to claim that the sceptic cares little about basing a system of philosophy upon a particular thing or grasping the whole through a certain part. Scepticism, Hegel ventures, is the negative side of the knowledge of the Absolute, and as such it presupposes reason, the positive side.[77]

Hegel's claim warrants further consideration. It is not readily apparent how the scepticism of Plato or of Homer is a negative aspect of the knowledge of the Absolute. Especially in the case of Homer it would seem that the art of portraying a given thing in manifold form is simply a renunciation of the Absolute. But, if such art is taken in the sense of speculation, as the ongoing attempt to portray things in the round, as it were, or to capture them in their totality by depicting them in their various poses, it becomes clear that Homer's manifold of appearances is united in its absolute totality. Or to put it somewhat differently, the dissimilarity of the various depictions of a given thing presupposes the absolute unity that is positively grasped by reason. This is all the clearer in the case of Plato, for he advocates a theory of absolute forms of which transitory phenomena are distinct representations.[78] Thus, according to Hegel, the scepticism of Plato and Homer alike, as well as that of the great Eleatic, Parmenides, was meant to question the reality of empirical consciousness, and this in the service of reason.[79]

Hegel extrapolates from Diogene's original insight by claiming that scepticism is implicit in every genuine philosophical system. Indeed such scepticism is the "free side" of such philosophical systems, whereby the basic concepts that comprise the system are taken up in their internal relation in a given proposition of reason:

> When that which is reflected upon itself isolates the concepts contained in any proposition that expresses reasonable knowledge, and the form in which they are joined is considered, then it must become evident that these concepts are cancelled and preserved, or are unified in such a way that they contradict one another. (Ibid. p. 231)[80]

In order to render Hegel's point more cogent it is necessary to see that the basic concepts which comprise a genuine system of philosophy are themselves manifold representations of the unity of reason. One must be careful then to distinguish this use of the term, concept (*Begriff*), from the later and more famous use of that term by Hegel in his mature philosophy. That a concept is here an empirical phenomenon of consciousness is clear from what Hegel says regarding ancient scepticism in passages later in the article.[81] If the concepts of a system of philosophy are taken as empirical phenomena, it is understandable how Hegel can present scepticism as the free side of systematic philosophy. The sceptical impulse is to find that the individual concepts of a given proposition are all at the same time cancelled, or otherwise combined such that they contradict one another. It is clear that Hegel is here employing a dialectical conception of reason, as presented, for example, in Kant's *Critique of Pure Reason*. Reason is conceived as that mode of thinking, which, when considered from a sceptical standpoint, results in the appearance of contradictions between the basic concepts of a proposition.

As an example of such a proposition Hegel considers Spinoza's claim that a cause is that which includes its existence within its essence, or that the nature of which can only be conceived of as existing.[82] The sceptical attitude sees in this proposition the following contradiction: the concept of essence or nature can be posited only insofar as existence is abstracted from it.[83] In Homer and in Plato, as in all others mentioned as genuinely sceptical thinkers, the essentiality of a given, existing phenomenon is denied, just as the givenness or existence of an essence is denied. Thus essence is determinable only as the opposition of existence, and existence as the opposition of essence. If the two are taken together, they must be so taken as to comprise a contradiction. Both are at once negated.

To further elaborate this point Hegel considers another example from Spinoza, i.e., that God is the immanent rather than the transcendent cause of the world.[84] The sceptical insight into the proposition that God is one with the world renders the proposition self-contradictory (because the cause is cause only insofar as it is opposed to the effect). Thereby the concepts of God as cause and the world as effect are cancelled. The antinomy of the one and the many is taken in the same vein by Spinoza: unity is posited as identical with multiplicity, and substance as identical with its attributes.[85] The sceptic takes this to mean that the concepts contradict one another. God is cause, and God is not cause; God is one, and God is not one; God is many, and not many; God has an essence that perishes:

> ... [God] has an essence which itself again perishes, etc., because essence is only conceivable in opposition to form, and form must be posited as identical with essence. (Ibid. p. 232)

In this the truth of scepticism is discovered, namely, that one word lies equally opposite all words: *pantei logoi logos isos antikeitai*. And from this truth is won a great insight into the nature of reason. The principle of contradiction is infringed upon in every proposition of reason.[86] Since the principle of contradiction is eternally cancelled and preserved in every true system, scepticism lies at the heart of philosophy:

> Since every genuine philosophy has this negative side, or eternally cancels the principle of contradiction, whoever has the urge can draw out this negative side directly, and produce it from any scepticism. (Ibid. p. 232f.)

Hegel's insight into the relation of scepticism and philosophy indicates that he has brought an emergent notion of dialectical thinking into play in this article, and one which has its origin in the doubleness of propositions formed in language. In the above passage Hegel suggested that the principle of contradiction lies implicit within every true philosophy, and in such a way that it can always be cancelled from the side of scepticism or preserved by formal reason. The term he uses to express this double possibility is the famous *aufheben*. In the relation between philosophy and scepticism the senses of *aufheben* as both "to cancel" and "to preserve" are held together in their absolute, or properly speculative form. Or to put it differently, speculation can always bring contradiction to speech in a philosophically constructive way. As much will become clear in the following consideration of the relation of genuine scepticism to the philosophy of reflection.

Hegel takes the Platonic philosophy as an example of a philosophy that embraces the knowing of reason. In so doing he has to enter into the ancient dispute over whether Plato was a dogmatic philosopher or a sceptic.[87] The influence of Sextus was decisive in presenting this struggle to posterity, and he designated Plato's philosophy as dogmatism. This led to a scepticism which sets itself against the reality of the Idea, or reason.

Hegel scrutinizes Sextus's treatment of reason. According to Sextus the claim of dogmatic philosophy is that reason knows itself through itself (*hoti oude heautes epignomon estin he dianoia, ho noos heauton katlambanetai*). Hegel notes that he attacks this claim in the following manner:

> If reason comprehends itself, either it must be *the whole* which comprehends itself, insofar as it comprehends itself, or it must employ, not the whole, but only a part for this [end]. Now, if it is the whole which comprehends itself, then the whole is comprehension and that which comprehends; but if the whole is that which comprehends, then there remains nothing left over to be comprehended. But it is completely unreasonable that comprehension should be, but not that which is comprehended. And also reason can not use a part of itself for this [end]; for how should the part comprehend itself? If it is a whole, then nothing remains for that which comprehends; if again with a part, how should this comprehend itself yet again, and so on into infinity; so that comprehension is without a principle, for either no first [principle] is found which deals with comprehension, or that which is supposed to be comprehended is nothing. (Ibid. p. 238)

Hegel notes that Sextus hereby presents the self-knowledge of reason as a radically subjective affair. Sextus then attempts to divide and conquer dogmatic philosophers by displaying their reliance upon a subjective conception of reason.[88] And once scepticism has thus torn itself away from reason, according to Hegel, it can take either of two forms, directing itself against reason, or not against it.[89]

To account for the path taken by scepticism in antiquity, Hegel considers the seventeen tropes of scepticism, as presented by Sextus. Without going through the treatment of each trope, one can note that Hegel takes the first ten to be directed, not against reason, but against the dogmatism of common consciousness, or empirical consciousness itself.[90] This class of scepticism is characterized by an *epoche* of consciousness, or the doubting of all things as well as the fact of consciousness itself. None of these first ten tropes, therefore, touch upon the matter of reason and its knowing. They address much rather only the finite and the knowledge of the finite, namely, understanding. The tropes are thus empirical in kind, and not speculative. As such this class of scepticism is not directed against reason and philosophy.[91]

What the first ten tropes of scepticism discover in a positive sense is the difference itself between appearance and concepts. This, according to Hegel, can facilitate the emergence of genuine philosophy, for the first step to be taken by philosophy is to realize the irreality and untruth of knowledge based in appearance.[92] It is also the basis of the sceptic's way of life. For the sceptic pursued a path of imperturbability (*ataraxia*) by denying that the appearance of disturbances (*tarache*) held any genuine truth.[93] Hegel notes in this context that philosophy and stoicism alike are rooted in this scepticism.[94] Pyrrho founded a school in this connection. But the school became fragmented, and scepticism directed itself in turn against dogmatism and philosophy.

According to Hegel, the final five tropes[95] of scepticism present powerful criticisms of the dogmatism of appearances, but do not directly engage philosophy itself. With regard to the former, these tropes give rise to insoluble antinomies. But with regard to the latter, such antinomies are transformed in the service of reason.[96] These tropes rely, in Hegel's estimation, upon reason[97] and yet reason itself can in turn be affected by them:

> Thus, since all of these tropes include in themselves the concept of a finite thing, and since they ground themselves upon this, through their use it happens that that which is reasonable is immediately turned into a finite something; in order to be able to scratch they furnish the itch of limitation. They do not in and of themselves oppose reasonable thinking, but when they do oppose it, as even Sextus uses them to do, they immediately alter the reasonable. (Ibid. p. 250)

Having considered ancient scepticism and its influence upon reason, Hegel essays to delineate the difference between it and the modern scepticism represented in Schulze's work. He rehearses the three basic forms of ancient scepticism:

> ... [ancient scepticism] is identical with philosophy, and only its negative side; or it is divorced from it, without being turned against it; or it is turned against it. (Ibid. p. 252)

Common to these three types of scepticism, Hegel reminds, is their orientation against the dogmatism of common consciousness. This, he avers, is what modern scepticism lacks.[98]

The emergence of this form of scepticism in modern times is, in Hegel's judgment, a unique development in the history of thought. He describes the project of modern scepticism as the denial of reason, and the transformation of the knowledge of the Absolute into finite knowing.[99] The foundation of modern scepticism is thus the rejection of the identity of thinking and being. This transformation of reason into reflection is worthy of consideration:

> The all-penetrating fundamental form of this transformation consists, however, in the fact that the contrary of the first definition of Spinoza (considered above as defining a *causa sui* as that which comprehends its essence at once with its existence) renders it a principle and determines the thought as an absolute fundamental proposition, which, because it is something thought, does not at once encompass a *being* within it. (Ibid. p. 253f.)

In particular, Hegel presses, the opposition of thinking and being known to the understanding has become entrenched in the rejection of the ontological proof for the existence of God[100]:

> The affirmation of this opposition is contrary to the so-called ontological proof for the existence of God, most foolishly and with infinite smugness; and as reflective judgment it appears in opposition to nature; and particularly in the form of a refutation of the ontological proof it has won a general and broad fame. (Ibid. p. 254f.)

In concluding his remarks on this matter, Hegel claims that modern scepticism is ultimately but a form of the Kantian philosophy.[101] And, because he thus identifies modern scepticism with Kantianism, we may justifiably skip over Hegel's detailed criticism of Schulze's scepticism. The analysis serves only to associate this scepticism with the fundamental principles and errors of Kant's philosophy of the understanding:

It is the spirit of Kantian philosophy to have consciousness of this highest idea[102] but to intentionally destroy it again. Thus we distinguish two spirits that are apparent in Kantian philosophy, one belonging to philosophy (which is always brought to ruin by the system) and another, belonging to the system, which proceeds from the death of the Idea of Reason. (Ibid. p. 272)

What is most clearly evoked by Hegel's hyperbole is the death of speculative reason. And it is this death which gives this treatment of scepticism its systematic tie to his next article, faith and knowledge.

In conclusion allow me to summarize the preceding and draw out the implications of the present article for the project at hand. Hegel's remarkable treatment of Schulze's new scepticism takes the reader well beyond anything presented in the previous article on Krug. Krug was the object of Hegel's critical remarks because he had proffered a system of philosophy devoid of any substantial sense of reason. And many of the same notes are sounded in the article on Schulze. But in Schulze's position Hegel found a far more worthy adversary. The new scepticism, like Krug's philosophy, based itself in an empiricist positivism, but, unlike Krug's, this philosophy set out to extirpate any and all traces of reason. Thus the modern sceptic, cheered on by the proponents of common sense philosophy, attacked speculative philosophy and its claims regarding reason and the Absolute. It did not simply render reason ineffectual by assigning it a minimal role in the theory of cognition, but went so far as to demonstrate that all claims made by reason, most especially that wherein God is said to exist according to his essence, were self-contradictory and otherwise blatantly opposed to what experience teaches.

Hegel responded to the challenge of modern scepticism by refining his notion of criticism (that to read philosophy means to see in every philosophical work the greater or lesser presentation of the one true philosophy) to include all opposition to philosophy as such. Criticism must take as its object also those works which are greater or lesser versions of the active opposition to the philosophy of reason. Criticism, then, essays not only to articulate the rift between common human understanding and philosophy proper, but also that between the common character of sceptical doubt and the seemingly contradictory claims of speculative reason. Accordingly, the view of the proponents of commonness in thinking as well as that of the common people in general is less that they are naive than that they are somewhat viciously so. For, in considering not only the historical origins of scepticism in Western antiquity, but also its source in the human attitudes of doubt and fear, Hegel exposed the penchant of doubters for the crassest nihilism. Nihilism because they rejected the claims of reason to grasp the Absolute as the identity of thinking and being. Crass because they did so by advancing a crude if hollow self-certainty in judgments about appearances.

To Hegel, the leaders and followers of modern scepticism were lacking in the nerve of the ancients to doubt the truth and reality of appearances as such, even as they were also without the courage to venture forth in speculation. And, by identifying this modern movement with the fundamental disinclination both to thus doubt and to think speculatively expressed in the *Critique of Pure Reason*, Hegel saw how Kant paled by comparison to a thinker such as Plato or Spinoza. For, though sceptical with regard to appearances, these thinkers were yet genuinely bold speculative philosophers of reason.

How paltry, then, must Kant's famous slogan, *Sapere aude!*[103] have seemed to the young critical thinker. Surely it was no slight matter for one who had previously embraced and lauded the efforts of Kant, as had Hegel, to now turn upon his former inspiration for being weak and hypocritical. How daring is a knowing which rejects the unity of thinking and being?

One can glean from Hegel's article on scepticism many important comments attesting to his growing seriousness as a thinker as well as to a mounting sense of dread and irony with regard to the attempt to think in an age that had turned its back upon philosophy. It should also be noted that Hegel's original insight into the speculative language of contradiction served an important if largely implicit role here.

In the opening passages of the present article Hegel remarked that scepticism must be scrutinized if one is to discover when it is more reasonable to doubt something than to dogmatically affirm it.[104] A more daunting task would be hard to find for a young thinker. For it is a root question of philosophy, to inquire what ought to be thought and what should be set aside as inimical to thought. Hegel, as we have seen, does not choose the easier path of garnishing his judgments on the matter with citations of the most influential authorities of the day. Nor does he take the next easiest path in accepting modern epistemological theory as the sole criterion by which to decide what can be known and what cannot, as Kant himself had done. Rather Hegel opts for the long and tortuous route of considering what philosophy and its companion turned nemesis, scepticism, have deemed necessary in the history of thinking and doubting and what can be said on this subject. Thus Hegel's extensive treatment of the origin and development of scepticism is no mere pretext. It is much rather, as he himself puts it, to ponder the negative side of the one true philosophy emergent in Western culture. In his new career as a speculative thinker, he shuns the characteristic philosophical and political *apragmosyne* of the day and its tendency to bury the history of philosophy beneath the overriding concerns of common sense and consensus regarding practical affairs.

The common error, alleged by Schulze to be the source of the late philosophical disharmony, was, in Hegel's critical view, not the cause but a symptom of the pervasive philosophical malaise.[105] The true cause of this condition was the philosophical failure of nerve to take up with the task of speculative reason, and to communicate its truth and reality to the people.[106]

The antinomies of reason, as recently presented in Kant's theoretical philosophy, were not to be taken, in Hegel's view, as the ultimate collapse of reason, but the transition from human understanding to human reason, which had its source in the spirit of ancient scepticism. And, if reason had to go under, because of the pressures put upon it by the late hegemony of the understanding, it had to do so only so that it could rise again in purified form. For the failure of reason in theoretical philosophy was but a part of the total collapse of thinking, theoretical, practical, and aesthetic alike. The true fate of speculative reason in this day was that it had to undergo a total destruction in the categories of the understanding, if later it was to emerge as the positive side of the negative impulse of scepticism. It had to be seen that the many and various failures of philosophy in its theoretical, practical, and aesthetic spheres were indeed united in the idea of a unified speculative thinking. The discovery of this fate and one's submission to it in thought had to be taken as a moment of critical thinking which strove to become fully and properly speculative.[107]

The claim of the modern sceptic was that speculation itself could not be grasped. But, Hegel maintained, that if we can at least see that the understanding sorts and arranges the facts of consciousness, as in the philosophy of Kant, we must just as surely be able to grasp reason as the self-knowledge of this process; if this cannot be taken as true and certain, nothing can.[108] He also exposed the inconsistency of the modern sceptic who, claiming that things exist with absolute certainty, would deny that they can be grasped by reason as they exist in themselves.[109]

Hegel maintained that we must at least begin with the ancient sceptic's doubt of the existence of the things of appearance.[110] And further we must see that this doubt is the negative side of the speculative grasp of the Absolute.[111] To recognize that this genuine scepticism is the negative side of reason is to begin to see reason in its truly speculative, dialectical totality.[112]

Hegel thus advanced that scepticism is implicit in every true philosophical system. He pointed out that the propositions of reason could always be brought to light as self-contradictory antinomies, as has occurred with the ontological proof of the existence of God. But, if taken in relation to reason, such contradiction could become manifest as the first step of speculative thought. Thus, that God is cause and not cause; one and not one; many and not many; that God has an essence which passes away in existence--these are the first expressions of speculative reason, the one word which lies equally opposite many words. Hegel proffered this speculative principle of contradiction as the truth of reason, eternally cancelled and preserved in every true philosophy.[113]

What the critic, what the speculative thinker, essayed to evoke was that philosophical *apragmosyne* had become the triumphant and universal fate of thinking, and that this fate entailed nothing less than the death of speculative reason.[114] For in this the critical speculative thinker attempted to sweep away the stoic hypocrisy of modern scepticism, leaving us to consider the act of killing the idea of reason, that idea which in being thought necessarily is.[115]

In the chapter to follow we will examine Hegel's treatment of this act of reflection under the aegis of the death of God.

ENDNOTES

[1]The original advertisement for the piece began as follows: *Kritisches Journal der Philosophie herausgegeben von F.W.J. Schelling und G.W.F. Hegel.* See Hartmut Buchner, *"Hegel und das Kritische Journal der Philosophie,"* Hegel-Studien 3 (1965) p. 95.

[2]See Buchner's and Pöggeler's appendix to GW Vol. 4, p. 540ff.

[3]See ibid., pp. 540-48.

[4]Night, pp. xxiiif, xlvi.

[5]See GW Vol. 4, pp. 533-37. The journal was from beginning to end Schelling's idea.

[6]Ibid. p. 534f.

[7]Ibid.

[8]Ibid. p. 535f.

[9]As we have seen, the fount of criticism re-emerged in the *Differenz* essay, and now it became a raging torrent.

[10]SW Vol. 1, p. 176.

[11]Ibid. p. 187.

[12]Ibid. p. 187f.

[13]Ibid. p. 173.

[14]Ibid. p. 175.

[15]That Hegel's choice of example is perspicuous is clear from his conception of philosophy as the pursuit of the Absolute, wherein God and nature are thought in their primordial unity.

[16]As this material has never been published in translation, I have offered my own.

[17]The affinities between these passages and those in the *Differenz* essay on the need of philosophy are clear, even down to the general division I presented in the language of pre-reflective, reflective, and post-reflective thinking.

[18]Ibid. p. 180.

[19]Ibid. p. 177.

[20]Ibid. p. 178.

[21]Ibid.

[22]The best example of this is the philosophy of Kant, for his works portray a vigorous critical spirit which scrutinizes the assumptions, conclusions, and practices of the entire Enlightenment.

[23]To use the example of Kant again, Hegel is referring to the extreme curtailment of the scope of reason and the limitation of its role in philosophy witnessed in the *Critique of Pure Reason*.

[24]Ibid. p. 179.

[25]Ibid. p. 185.

[26]The division between consciousness and its object characteristic of this philosophy rendered the objectivity of thinking suspect, and so led to a kind of subjectivism. Thought was conceived of along the lines of a faculty of the understanding --the activity of the mind in abstraction from its object-- rather than as that unity of mind and object known as reason.

[27]Kant is surely not to be excluded here. His philosophy fits under the general heading of Cartesianism. It is but a one-sided form of Descartes's dualism of mind and body. For the Kantian philosophy is the working out of Descartes's system exclusively from the side of the *cogito*. In Kant the mind does not posit the body, but rather the limitation of mind known in experience.

[28]Hegel nowhere states such a principle of reading. However, some such hermeneutical notion is implicit and effective in all of his philosophical criticism. For he reads the history of thought as a grand discourse on the as yet latent idea of philosophy. Thus all accounts of knowledge (what philosophy manifestly is) are rendered by Hegel as more or less incomplete and unreflective accounts of the self-knowledge of reason. This matter will become abundantly clear in the following discussion.

[29]We can only surmise here. Perhaps Hegel is referring to something like the naivete of Plato's slave boy, who in the *Meno* unreflectively expounds the profound truths of geometry. In any case, what seems to be essential to Hegel's notion of the 'beautiful soul' is the lack of reflectivity in thinking. For becoming reflective about thought leads initially only to confusion, just as in the folk-tale the centipede stumbled over how he was able to walk.

[30]By mixing these metaphors I have perhaps accorded too much to an implicit notion of resurrection. On the basis of the individual metaphors alone, this would be unwarranted. Both images suggest a recurrent cycle of life and death, and not the final transcendence of death through a superlative sort of life. However, if one were to reverse the priority, and read the resurrection in light of the other two images, the suggestion would be that the transcendent meaning of life is to die: the philosopher dies, but dies knowing death as the fate of the Absolute. However, this topic will be broached numerous times by Hegel in the discussions to follow, and so should not be pressed at this point.

[31]One certainly wonders how much Schelling recognized Hegel's project.

[32]Ibid. p. 181. Hegel's claim is odd, given that Locke and Hobbes are generally held to be the major voices in modern empiricism. Perhaps it is helpful to consider that Hegel wishes to emphasize how Kant seemingly superseded the British empiricists with his new empirical epistemology.

[33]This article was to appear with the material which preceded it in the first volume of the journal, but was too long, and so became the first part of the second volume. See *Jenaer Kritische Schriften II*; *Glauben und Wissen*, ed. Hans Brockard and Hartmut Buchner (Hamburg: Felix Meiner Verlag, 1982) p. xii. This indicates that there is perhaps a programmatic break between the article on faith and knowledge and that which follows it, on natural law. This latter article presents an application of the idea of philosophy to individual sciences, indicating that the idea itself had already been presented *in ovo*.

[34]Though he does not go as far as I have here, Harris notes the relation between the *Critical Journal* and the *Phenomenology*:

"In *Faith and Knowledge* the program [i.e., of the *Critical Journal*] was put into effect, over its whole range .... And it is not only the method but the matter which makes *Faith and Knowledge* a first sketch for that still unthought of major work [i.e., the Phenomenology]. *Faith and Knowledge* is Hegel's first attempt to survey the culture of the time, and to place all the signs of the advent of 'absolute knowledge' in an ideal context which would cause them to reveal their meaning." (*Faith and Knowledge*, p. 3f.)

[35]Kaufmann, *Hegel* p. 81f.
[36]SW Vol. 1, p. 195.
[37]Ibid. p. 195f.
[38]Ibid. p. 198.
[39]Ibid. p. 199.
[40]Ibid. p. 204f.
[41]Ibid. p. 205f.
[42]Ibid. p. 206.
[43]See ibid. pp. 200, 210ff.
[44]Ibid. p. 196.
[45]Ibid. p. 199.
[46]Ibid.
[47]Ibid. p. 205.
[48]Ibid.
[49]The paradoxical image employed here echoes the discussion in the *Differenzschrift* of the Absolute as both the conclusion and the presupposition of reason.
[50]Ibid. p. 212.
[51]Ibid. p. 199.
[52]Ibid. p. 200f.
[53]Ibid. p. 208f.
[54]Just what this philosophy might be is a matter of debate among scholars. Most especially scrutinized is the question whether Hegel refers here and in other like passages to his as yet unwritten philosophical system or to Schelling's philosophy. The matter cannot be decided here. However, as Masakatsu Fujita notes, the foundational conception of reason assumed here, i.e., that reason is the appearance of the Absolute, is uniquely Hegel's. Masakatsu Fujita, *Philosophie und Religion beim jungen Hegel, Hegel-Studien* p. 156f.
[55]SW Vol. 1, pp 213-275.
[56]The importance of this article is often overlooked. Yet here we find a decisive difference between Hegel and his colleague, Schelling. The point is related to that of Fujita, cited above. For just as essence and appearance must be said to belong to the Absolute in-itself, so too the Absolute must be seen to encompass the negation of its appearance within its very essence. This single idea will characterize the thought of the mature philosopher. An enlightening study on this topic is to be found in Michael N. Forster, *Hegel and Skepticism* (Cambridge, Massachusetts and London England: Harvard University Press, 1989).
[57]Ibid. p. 215f.
[58]As is clear from Hegel's commentary, Schulze refers to the Kantian philosophy here. See ibid. p. 215.
[59]Ibid.
[60]Ibid. p. 216f. Hegel's reference to such failed speculative pursuits is clearer when one bears in mind his criticism of Krug's charge that philosophy ought to be able to deduce the existence of

his feather pen. See the discussion above in this chapter's section on common sense.

[61]It is worth noting in passing that Hegel here identifies the death of speculative philosophy with the figure of Socrates, whereas in the next article, *Glauben und Wissen*, the identification is with Christ. As will be seen in the chapter to follow, there the matter is considered from without, as the external fate suffered by God and speculative reason. The crucial point here, however, is that common sense philosophy must bear the burden of the death of speculative thinking.

[62]As will become apparent in the chapter on the article on natural law, the implied comparison of the execution of Socrates and the death of a people is crucial to Hegel. The issue there, however, is considered from within, so that the death of a people is seen to be the highest expression of freedom in politics and philosophy. Just as Socrates once faced death, a people is now seen to risk itself in the form of speculative thinking. This is to comprehend from within what appears in the article on faith and knowledge as the external fate suffered by God. However, it must be stressed again that the point in the present article is that to philosophize according to common sense is to put speculative thought to death. Whether this entails the death of God and that of a people is not explicit.

[63]Ibid.

[64]Ibid. p. 219.

[65]For Hegel's description see ibid. p. 221.

[66]Ibid. p. 222.

[67]See ibid. p. 222f.

[68]It should not be overlooked that Hegel's presentation of the positive aspect of Schulze's scepticism is in effect to reduce that aspect to the common sense philosophy represented by Krug.

[69]See ibid. p. 225f. Presumably Schulze's theory of the priority of empirical consciousness precludes the notion of a pure science, such as mathematics.

[70]Ibid.

[71]Ibid. One might contrast the cynic, Diogenes of Sinope, who rejected the knowledge of appearance even to the point of trading practicality for his place in the sun.

[72]Ibid. p. 226f.

[73]Ibid. p. 227.

[74]Ibid. p. 229.

[75]Ibid. p. 230.

[76]As is clear from Chapter XXXVI of the *Republic*, Plato considers art in general to be a manipulation of the appearances of the empirical world. And, since art is an illusory representation of the already illusory experience of the senses, it is at the farthest remove from the truth of reason. However, this definition of art indicates that Plato saw clearly how the artist's manipulation of appearances is indeed a rejection of the truth of empirical reality.

[77]SW Vol. 1, p. 230f.

[78]See *Republic*, Chap. XIX.

[79]SW Vol. 1, p. 231.

[80]It is worthy of note that Hegel employs the term, *aufheben* (cancelled and preserved), here in the properly dialectical sense characteristic of his mature thought: the contradictions that arise through the concepts of the understanding are transformed in the propositions of reason. Another way of putting this is to say that concepts are understood in relation to other concepts, and especially so when they are in opposition. Forster has noted that Hegel adopted this notion of *equipollence* from ancient scepticism and fashioned it into an important basis for his epistemology. See *op. cit.*, pp. 3ff., 10, 174ff.

[81]See ibid. p. 243.

[82]Ibid. p. 231f.

[83]Ibid. p. 232.

[84]Ibid.

[85]Ibid.

[86]Ibid.

[87]Ibid. p. 236.

[88]See ibid. p. 238f. The point involves the ancient dispute as to the proper resting place of reason. Sextus maintains that if philosophers disagree as to whether reason resides, for example, in the head or the breast, etc. surely this is proof that wherever reason is said to reside it must be in subjectivity. That Hegel took Sextus's criticism quite seriously is attested by the long section devoted to physiognomy and phrenology in the *Phenomenology*. Here Hegel wrestles with the question of the proper resting-place of reason. See the section on Observing Reason.

[89]Ibid. p. 239f.

[90]Ibid. p. 241.

[91]Ibid. p. 242f. It is clear here that the present article on scepticism marks a progression from the previous consideration of common sense.

[92]Ibid. p. 243.

[93]Ibid. p. 245.

[94]Ibid. p. 243. It should be noted in passing that the relationship between scepticism and stoicism is treated in the same vein in the *Phenomenology* in the section on the freedom of self-consciousness.

[95]Hegel lists the tropes as follows: *Verschiedenheit, Unendliche, Verhältniss, Voraussetzung, Gegenseitige.* There remain two tropes identified by Sextus, but Hegel, following Diogenes, reduces them to instances of those that precede them. See ibid. p. 246f.

[96]Ibid. p. 247f.

[97]The matter is somewhat more involved than I have indicated here, but a thorough treatment would go beyond the scope of the present investigation.

[98]Ibid. p. 252f.

[99]Ibid.

[100]The reference is principally to Kant's treatment of this proof in the *Critique of Pure Reason* in the Transcendental Dialectic.

[101]SW Vol. 1, p. 256.

[102]The idea in question is that of reason. See ibid. p. 272.

[103]The slogan is from *What is Enlightenment?*

[104]See SW Vol. 1, p. 215.

[105]See ibid. p. 216.

[106]See ibid. p. 217.

[107]See ibid. p. 220.

[108]See ibid. p. 223.

[109]See ibid. p. 224.

[110]See ibid. p. 226.

[111]See ibid. p. 230.

[112]See ibid. p. 231.

[113]See ibid. p. 232.

[114]See ibid. p. 217.

[115]See ibid. p. 272.

5 | FAITH AND KNOWLEDGE

The next of Hegel's journal articles, and the most important for the present investigation, takes up where the discussion of scepticism left off. He argues that the philosophy of reflection stemming from Kant's writings constitutes the next step in the unfolding of knowledge. First came the philosophy of commmon sense and its naive empiricism. Then the new sceptical philosophy and its more complex grasp of empiricism. Now we shall see how consciousness turns away from the outside world in order to reflect on its own activity. But Hegel finds in the advance of knowledge a crisis for philosophy. He attempts in *Glauben und Wissen* to present the reflection-philosophy in its totality and to criticize it for its extreme subjectivism, a subjectivism which precludes access to the unity of being and thinking. It is this failure of philosophy which leads to the utterance of the death of God.

> But the pure concept of infinity as the abyss of nothingness in which all being is engulfed, must signify the infinite grief [of the finite] purely as a moment of the supreme Idea, and no more than as a moment. Formerly, the infinite grief only existed historically in the formative process of culture. It existed as the feeling that 'God Himself is dead.' upon which the religion of more recent times rests; the feeling that Pascal expressed in so to speak sheerly empirical form: *'la nature est telle qu'elle marque partout un Dieu perdu et dans l'homme et hors de l'homme.* [Nature is such that it *signifies* everywhere a lost God both within and outside man.] By marking this feeling as a moment of the supreme Idea, the pure concept must give philosophical existence to what used to be either the moral precept that we must sacrifice the empirical being (*Wesen*), or the concept of formal abstraction [e.g., the categorical imperative]. Thereby it must re-establish from philosophy the Idea of absolute freedom and along with it the absolute Passion, the speculative Good Friday in place of the historic Good Friday. Good Friday must be speculatively re-established in the whole truth and harshness of its

143

> Godforsakenness. Since the [more] serene, less well-grounded, and more individual style of the dogmatic philosophies and of the natural religions must vanish, the highest totality can and must acheive its resurrection soley from this harsh consciousness of loss, encompassing everything, and ascending in all its earnestness and out of its deepest ground to the most serene freedom of its shape.[1]

But this is to get ahead of matters. Let us back up to resume the train of thought initiated in the article on common sense.

Reflection-philosophy, like common sense and scepticism, has as its primary concern the fact and role of consciousness in human knowledge. However, unlike the other two, reflection-philosophy construes the relation of consciousness and its object in terms of opposition. The principal opposition is that between the percept and the concept. Despite this opposition, however, the philosophy of reflection aims finally at reconciling the empirical with the ideal and the practical with the theoretical. Hegel describes the situation to be overcome in the reflection-philosophy as follows. When considered from the perspective of theory, the empirical is nothing. This is scepticism. When viewed from the perspective of practice, however, the empirical is everything. This is common sense.[2] What Hegel is driving at is the unhappy relation between concept and intuition in Kantian philosophy. He knew well that neither the theoretical first *Critique* nor the practical second *Critique* adequately solved the problem of concept and intuition. This was nothing new on Hegel's part, as all of Kant's successors had recognized this fundamental problem. However, that reflection-philosophy is at once common sense empiricism and scepticism, at once positivism and nihilism, had escaped the notice of even its most astute representatives. Hegel therefore took it as his task in this article to expose the absolute opposition of these elements of the reflection-philosophy.

He depicts this opposition in terms of the finite, or the empirical, and the infinite, or the ideal. The identification of the finite with the empirical and the infinite with the ideal is in the philosophy of reflection weighted in favor of the empirical, and so the aspect of idealism and its conception of the Absolute is inadequate[3]. The consequence is a knowledge and a faith which fails to grasp the true subject of reason, namely, the Absolute.

Hegel demonstrates that the systems of Kant, Jacobi, and Fichte taken together represent the totality, or system, of the philosophy of reflection. Kant presents the objectivity of reflection-philosophy through his use of the concept as absolute; Jacobi represents the subjective side in the infinite yearning for the Absolute; Fichte provides a synthesis of the two by portraying a subjective identity between the objectivity of Kant and the subjectivity of Jacobi.[4]

In saying that Kant, Jacobi, and Fichte represent the totality of reflection-philosophy, Hegel lays claim to understanding the inherent relation between common sense and scepticism. The empirically based philosophy of reflection strives to reconcile the sceptical antinomy of concepts and common sense consciousness in the form of a subjective idealism. The attempt does not meet with success; the subjectivity of Fichte's synthesis of the (sceptical) Kantian and the (common sensical) Jacobian systems is reducible to a basic truth of the philosophy of reflection: thinking which begins with the empirical cannot escape the empirical, and especially not by way of a problematic notion of the reasonable and the Absolute. This becomes in its highest form the incompleteness of thought[5]. However, the union of common sense and scepticism manifest in the reflection-philosophy as the incompleteness of thinking marks the climax of a world-spiritual principle. To anticipate this may be called the death of God.

We turn now to the argument itself. Hegel's article begins by reflecting upon the age-old distinction between faith and reason. According to Hegel, this distinction had in recent culture finally found its way into reflection-philosophy in the modified form of an opposition between faith and knowledge.

Hegel's claim is that reason had won the day in this old struggle, and that consequently the problem of faith had been annexed by philosophy. In this way philosophy established its autonomy and independence from religion. Nevermore would reason be called the handmaid of faith[6].

Yet Hegel remarked something curious in this victory. So decisive was reason's conquest of faith that it was no longer correct to speak of a conflict between them. In fact reason had laid such a great claim upon faith that religion had become dependent upon philosophy for explicating the grounds of its articles of faith. But in this Hegel unearthed a grand contradiction. Philosophy had triumphed over religion only to fall in turn to the vanquished[7]. The struggle between philosophy and religion had resulted, according to Hegel, in both being radically transformed. Most importantly, the philosophy of understanding had placed reason out of its reach and over against itself in a weakened form of faith. The eternal was beyond the grasp of this Enlightenment philosophy:

> Thus what used to be regarded as the death of philosophy, that Reason should renounce its existence in the Absolute, excluding itself totally from it and relating itself to it only negatively, became now the zenith of philosophy. By coming to consciousness of its own nothingness, the Enlightenment turns this nothingness into a system. (Ibid. p. 56)

The failure of Enlightenment philosophy lies, according to Hegel, in its incompleteness, its inability to include reason within its systems. But this incompleteness is, as we have seen, itself the completion, the coming to consciousness and development, of a form of the world-spirit. Hegel dubs this form the principle of the North, of Protestantism.[8]

This principle is the subjectivity in which are expressed beauty and truth, feeling and sentiment, love and understanding. Yet it is a form of subjectivity so extreme that it amounts to a crisis of world consciousness. It is a debilitating form of subjectivism, according to which the objective and external is null. He characterizes the Protestant principle's attitude toward objectivity as follows:

> That beauty should become real in objective form, and fall captive to objectivity, that consciousness should seek to be directed at exposition and objectivity themselves, that it should want to shape appearance or, shaped in it, to be at home there--all this should cease; for it would be a dangerous superfluity, and an evil, as the intellect could turn it into a thing (*zu einem Etwas*). (Ibid. p. 57)

But, Hegel insists, the power of the understanding to do just this --to turn the grove to lumber, the image to thing, beauty to fiction--is a necessary element of the principle of Protestantism.[9] Hegel's exposition is terse here, but he seems to refer to a pietistic philosophy with a bad conscience: subjectivity flees the finite, yearning for the infinite, but, because infinity is beyond its reach, it returns to finitude, embracing it in the understanding. Thus the philosophy of the Enlightenment exploits the flight of pietism in its theory of the understanding: subjectivity is presented as contingent upon finite objects, because consciousness is consciousness of finitude and the empirical. Thus Enlightenment philosophy pulls a metaphysical switch on Protestant subjectivity, replacing its unattainable object of desire, the Absolute, with the object of finite knowledge. But pietism is susceptible to this trick because of its fear of objectifying the Absolute. And so the world-spirit is, in Hegel's estimation, ship-wrecked upon the shores of the empirical.

Hegel focuses on the aim of piety in order to expose an important possibility for knowledge. The pure subjectivity of Protestantism is, as feeling, still a yearning for what is real and true, namely, the eternal and Absolute.[10] To resist the temptation of Enlightenment philosophy to absolutize the finite object is to reveal another and more genuine path to knowledge. If the longing of subjectivity were to attain its object, it would be transformed into a temporal beauty which is the fulfillment of worldly beings:

> But [what the longing does not recognize is that] when empirical existence is the pure body of inward beauty, it ceases to be something temporal and on its own. (Ibid. p. 57)

Here the the individual would not be a single thing alone unto itself. The individual would here be fulfilled; its yearning for the Absolute would attain complete intuition and blissful delight. Hegel does not pursue the ideal of the pure body of inner beauty at this juncture, however.[11] Instead he turns his attention to the philosophy of reflection, to the failure of that ideal.

With the advent of the Enlightenment, the infinite yearning of the body for something beyond the world reconciled itself with the empirical existence of the self. But this only in a failed sense. The reconciliation of self and its object of yearning was effected only through the reality of the empirical world being accepted by subjectivity as its objectivity. Thus this reconciliation was not that of the absolute opposition belonging to beatific yearning, but was instead merely one between the self and the world. The result was that the unconscious certainty of sinking into empirical existence had to be justified by the fact of the necessity of nature, and this bolstered by the notion of a good conscience.[12]

This failed reconciliation of consciousness is developed in the doctrine of happiness, so that the empirical subject and the common actuality with which it is reconciled can be grasped in confidence, without the stain of sin. According to Hegel, this doctrine was embodied in the philosophy of the understanding.[13] But, Hegel argues, the dogmatism of the Enlightenment and eudaemonism does not raise happiness to the highest level, making of it an idea. This would be to render it free of anything empirical, arbitrary, and sensual. In highest existence reasonable action and superlative bliss are one, so that it is a matter of indifference whether such existence be taken from the side of its ideality (reasonable action) or its reality (bliss and feeling). Here reality and ideality mutually condition one another: the highest happiness is the highest idea. But in the philosophy of the Enlightenment the reality and the ideality of existence are divorced, and the former (bliss and feeling) is posited as absolute existence.

When this philosophy came to dominate the age, the finite emerged as the sole reality, with the concept of happiness posed over and against it as the condition of this reality.[14] Thus eternity was denied any genuine existence. The eternal is here an unknowable God who lies on the far side of the limits of reason. And, Hegel concludes, because intuition and bliss are here empirically conceived, neither do they provide access to this God. Hegel describes the fundamental tendency of this cultural development as follows:

> This is the basic character of eudaemonism and the Enlightenment. The beautiful subjectivity of Protestantism is transformed into empirical subjectivity; the poetry of Protestant grief that scorns all reconciliation with empirical existence is transformed into the prose of satisfaction with the finite and of good conscience about it. (Ibid. p. 61)

The transformation of the poetry of grief into the prose of contentment occurs, according to Hegel, without the conscious intention of the representative thinkers of the Enlightenment. Indeed the express aim of the philosophies of Kant, Jacobi, and Fichte is to steer clear of eudaemonism and the trappings of empirical happiness. So much is this the case, however, that their philosophies represent only a modification of eudaemonism. For, even though these thinkers struggle constantly against eudaemonism, this is their sole opponent, and thus the condition of their every move.[15] Being thus enthralled by the doctrine of empirical happiness, Enlightenment philosophy brings to completion a development which has nothing to do with reason as such. But, if the conscious opposition of Enlightenment philosophy to eudaemonism can be seen as an unconscious affinity between the two, then the possibility arises of revealing an absolute opposition between the empirical and the Absolute. If further it can be shown that the concept of happiness in Enlightenment philosophy is nothing but the empirical happiness of eudaemonism, then the shortcoming of the concepts of understanding as such becomes apparent. For here it is seen that the concept is at once the conscious opposition to the empirical and the unconscious affinity with the empirical. This inherent division of the concept displays that the empirical is for it at once absolute reality and nothing.

The opposition of absolute empirical reality and nothing, however, marks the first step of reflection in philosophy.[16] For here it is clear that on one hand the concept is the ideality of empirical reality, and on the other it is wholly devoid of such reality. When the concept is the ideality of empirical reality, we have common sense empiricism. When it is devoid of empirical reality, we have scepticism. The former is the possibility of practical philosophy and the latter is the impossibility of theoretical philosophy.

By pressing the opposition between empirical, practical philosophy and non-empirical, theoretical philosophy, Hegel exposes the shortcoming of both. For practical philosophy is made out to be mere eudaemonism, and theoretical philosophy is shown to be nothing at all. Faced with this dilemma, Hegel urges the need for reworking theoretical philosophy. Without an adequate theoretical philosophy, we are fated to accept the absolute reality of eudaemonism, a reality which precludes the true reconciliation of empirical existence and the eternal Absolute.

Once Hegel has established that the fundamental principle of the North and of Protestantism is the absoluteness of the finite, and thus also the absolute contradiction of the finite and the infinite, of reality and ideality, the sensuous and the super-sensuous, and the otherworldliness of the genuinely real and Absolute, he is prepared to argue that the Kantian, Jacobian, and Fichtean philosophies represent the totality of this principle. He avers that the Kantian philosophy presents the infinite concept (the non-empirical concepts of understanding) as the sole objectivity of philosophical knowledge. Jacobi's philosophy proffers the infinite subjectivity of instinct, drive, and individuality. Fichte displays the infinite subjectivity, as objectified in obligation (*Sollen*) and striving. Thus Kant's infinite objectivity of knowledge is opposed by Jacobi's infinite subjectivity of feeling, and both are synthesized in Fichte's infinity of feeling become obligation.

Together these philosophical systems consciously express the sole concern of overcoming the eudaemonism of the subjective and the empirical, and vindicating the absoluteness and unconditionedness of reason by common actuality. But, because all alike conceive of reason as merely directed away from the empirical, the infinity of reason lies only in its relation to the finite. Thus they remain in the sphere of empirical finitude. All have failed to attain the Idea.

The failed attempt to transcend the empirical element of knowing and doing, as represented in Kant, Jacobi, and Fichte, is, in Hegel's judgment, the raising of reflection-culture to the level of a system. This culture is one which aims at elevating common human understanding to universal thinking. But, because of the form of thought this culture employs, it is denied any intuition of the eternal. The infinite concept is devoid of eternal intuition. The agony of those suffering under this limitation, or absolute opposition, expresses itself in the yearning and striving of a consciousness which cannot overcome itself. That consciousness is displayed in a faith in the beyond, but as a perennial incapacity and impossibility to attain what is beyond it.[17]

The philosophy which guides the culture of reflection is incapable of knowing God, according to Hegel, and so turns instead toward human being:

> This so-called man and his humanity conceived as a rigidly, insuperably finite sort of Reason form [Enlightenment][18] philosophy's absolute standpoint. Man is not a glowing spark of eternal beauty, or a spiritual focus of the universe, but an absolute sensibility. He does, however, have the faculty of faith so that he can touch himself up here and there with a spot of alien supersensuousness. (Ibid. p. 65)

Thus, Hegel holds, Enlightenment philosophy occupies itself not with the idea of human being, but with an abstraction of a humanity enmeshed in the limitations of the empirical, "impaled on the stake of the absolute antithesis."

The Enlightenment philosophy, according to Hegel, cuts itself off from the whole by fixating upon the absoluteness of the finite. If instead the Absolute were grasped from out of the unity of the finite and the infinite, the abstraction of the finite, as truth and reality, would pass away. This is to negate what is in itself the negation of the Absolute, and so is itself true affirmation.[19]

To fail to accomplish this is at once to embrace pure negation and pure position. But this is to pose thinking and being against each other, to pit absolute ego against absolute thing. It is with a view to this discontinuity of thinking and being in the culture of eudaemonism and enlightenment that Hegel scrutinizes the respective philosophies of Kant, Jacobi, and Fichte.

A. *Kant*

Hegel's basic criticism of Kant's philosophy of reflection is that it conceives of the Absolute as a mere subjective postulate, rather than as the sole proper, objective content of philosophy. Regarding this critical idealism, Hegel remarks the following:

> The highest Idea which it encountered in is critical business [i.e., the Idea of God in the Ontological Argument] it treated at first as if it were empty musing, nothing but an unnatural scholastic trick for conjuring reality out of concepts. Then in the final stage of its development, Kant's philosophy establishes the highest Idea as a postulate which is supposed to have necessary subjectivity, but not that absolute objectivity which would get it recognized as the only starting point of philosophy and its sole content instead of being the point where philosophy terminates in faith. (Ibid. p. 67)

Because of the status of the Absolute in his philosophy, Kant presents a critical idealism which limits the standpoint of philosophy to the unity of reflection. Hegel does not at this point venture an explanation of the term, *Reflexion*, but it stems from a section of Kant's *Critique of Pure Reason*. Kant describes reflection as asking the following question: In which of our cognitive faculties are our representations connected together? Is it the understanding, or is it the senses, by which they are combined or compared?[20] According to this definition the problem of reflection involves, not only the sorting of various representations according to their respective cognitive sources, but also the task of grasping those sources together in their unity. It is this latter question which most directly concerns Hegel, for his contention is that Kant conceives of the unity of understanding and sensation subjectively, from the side of understanding. This, he argues, is to settle upon a merely subjective resolution to the opposition between understanding and sensation. This in turn is tantamount to conceding that the opposition is finally unresolvable in a rigorous sense, and so signals a limitation in human knowledge.

Therefore, in Hegel's somewhat paradoxical way of putting it, the Kantian philosophy makes this opposition the absolute end of philosophy: it is the pure limit and thus the negation of philosophy.[21]

According to Hegel, if Kant's philosophy makes the opposition of sensation and understanding the absolute end and limit of knowledge, then surely it cannot share with genuine philosophy the attempt to resolve this opposition and such related ones as those between spirit and world, soul and love, ego and nature, etc. The sole idea of philosophy, Hegel maintains, is the transcendence of opposition in absolute identity. This is neither the universal, subjective, unrealizable postulate, nor that faith which lies beyond knowledge. Of course, for Kant, it was both.

Though Kant did not share this notion of philosophy, according to Hegel, his thought implied as much, even if only against its own intention. For Kant's philosophy brought fundamental oppositions to the fore in conspicuous form. His antinomies of the *Critique of Pure Reason* immediately draw attention to the rudimentary tensions in his thought. Hegel latched onto this element of Kantian philosophy, and exploited it through underscoring the subjectivity of Kant's idealism.

Kant's philosophy is clearly idealism, Hegel argues, because it asserts that the concept alone and intuition alone are nothing, and thus that their identity in experience is not an object of reason. But Kant's philosophy professes that experience is the only genuine form of knowledge, and that it alone can serve theoretical and practical reason. This, for Hegel, is its subjectivity. Just why Hegel claims Kant's notion of experience is subjective, however, must be spelled out in some detail.

Hegel's argument is based on the claim that Kant begins his philosophy with a conception of reason which ineluctably leads to a subjective account of experience.

Hegel's opinion is that Kant began well the task of philosophy, but ended poorly. The idea of reason is expressed in Kant's basic question: How are synthetic judgments possible *a priori*? But the Kantian philosophy fails to develop this question in its properly objective form:

> How are synthetic judgments *a priori* possible? This problem expresses nothing else but the Idea that subject and predicate of the synthetic judgment are identical in the *a priori* way. That is to say, these heterogeneous elements, the subject which is the particular and in the form of being, and the predicate which is the universal and in the form of thought, are at the same time absolutely identical. (Ibid. p. 69)

The possibility of this juxtaposition of such heterogenous elements is reason, the prior unity of those elements. Hegel identifies this unity in the Kantian notion of the original synthetic unity of apperception:

> This original synthetic unity must be conceived, not as produced out of opposites, but as a truly necessary, absolute, original identity of opposites. As such, it is the principle both of productive imagination, which is the unity that posits the difference as identical but distinguishes itself from the different. (Ibid. p. 70)

This in answer to Kant's notion of reflection: the faculties of understanding and sensation are not distinct origins of cognition, for both have their source in reason.

The truth of Kant's dictum that intuition without a concept is blind[22] attests to the unity of reason. For, according to Hegel, sensible intuition[23] taken on its own is sunken in the sheer difference of the sensations which comprise it. As such it does not distinguish itself as a unity from those sensations, for this distinction is the work of the understanding. The only unity belonging to sensible intuition is the sum total of those sensations which comprise its content. As Hegel puts it, identity in intuition is fully identical with difference.[24]

Here Hegel begins to push beyond Kant. For he proposes to answer why space and time are the only forms of sensible intuition: the identity of being and the identity of thinking correspond respectively to the Kantian pure forms of intuition, space and time.[25] By pressing this distinction, Hegel exposes a basic rift in the Kantian notion of intuition. This requires some explication. Hegel exploits the opposition in Kant's conception of intuition. That opposition is something like the following. If intuition is sensible, it must receive its object through the senses. The sensible form of intuition is to be distinguished from its intelligible form. If intelligible, intuition furnishes its own object, as, for example, language provides itself with meaning, or dreams create for themselves the images which make them up.[26] Sensible intuition, however, is not self-generative, but rather receptive.

Let us pause to reflect on sensible intuition. The receptivity of sensible intuition divides into contraries. We have, on one side, the intuition of the fragmentariness of sensation. The senses perceive detail for the sake of variety itself. This involves a certain lack of focus in one's perceptions, as, for example, when on a hot summer's afternoon one hears the far off rumble of a speeding train suddenly punctuated by the minute chirp of a cricket, and this followed immediately with every other little sound belonging to the world. On the other side is the intuition of the totality of sensation. The senses perceive the complete unity of the experience, as though one now encountered the train while standing on the tracks, at the point of impact. The experience is totalizing, unified in a way which precludes distinction or articulation of various sensations.

The underlying presence of these two sides of sensible intuition is expressed in Kant's use of the term, manifold, to denote the field of perception. For 'manifold' names at once the fragments and the totality of sensation. Hegel picks up on this, and describes Kant's manifold as comprised of the opposition of the identity of being and the identity of thinking. The step here is not an easy one to follow, but it involves taking being with the totality of sensation (e.g., the impact of the speeding train) and thinking with the fragments of sensation (e.g., the cricket's chirp, etc. above the rumbling of the train). The identity of being is the sheer inertia (rest in motion) of sensation. The identity of thinking is the discursiveness of sensation. This is why Hegel conjoins being and space, thinking and time. With this conjunction it becomes apparent that he is driving at an opposition which lies at the heart of Kant's analysis of the pure intuitions of space and time: so long as intuition is sensible, rather than intellectual, it will harbor within itself the contraries of space and time.

Hegel next sets the opposition within sensible intuition off against the concepts of the understanding. In so doing he again follows Kant initially. He invokes the other half of Kant's dictum: the concept without intuition is empty.[27] Thus emerges an opposition between concept and intuition.

In the case of the pure concepts of the understanding (which according to Kant are devoid of any elements of sensible intuition) Hegel maintains that we have the empty identity of being. Hegel formulates the matter thus:

> In isolation the pure concept is the empty identity. It is only as being relatively identical with that which it stands against, that it is concept; and it is [thus] plenished only through the manifold of intuition: sensuous intuition A = B, concept A2 = (A = B). (Ibid. p. 70f.)

Here we propose that A stands for the class of contraries including being and space, and B stands for the class comprising thinking and time. Thus it is apparent that the concept is the one-sided, empty, subjective identity of being and thinking, space and time. For the concept equals being and space, as opposed to intuition, which equals being, space, thinking, time.[28] The Kantian concept, then, is nothing but the abstract, universalized form of sensible intuition. This is the extent to which Kant's philosophy of the concepts of understanding is, according to Hegel, subjective and empty.

Two other matters lend support to this point. First, Hegel groups Kant's concept with the contraries subject/being/space.[29] This is because he takes the concept to be the abstract (formal) identity of the opposition which lies within opposition. Because the concept is the subjective identity of being, it is connected with space. Hegel calls the pure concept the empty identity of being. But, for Hegel, because the pure concept is abstracted from the manifold of intuition, it is as such empty. It thus stands in need of that to which it stands opposed, namely, sensible intuition.

Second, just as Kant's concept must be identified with the empty space of subjective being, so too intuition in the Kantian usage must be taken with the replete time of predicative thinking. In that the intuition is replete, it is in excess of the conceptual. As such Kant calls it blind.

This may require elaboration. The blindness of intuition is to be taken, not in the sense of the incapacity to see, but rather as the overwhelming of the faculty of vision by the panorama of sensible experience. Intuition is blinded by confusion. The threat that intuition might cause conceptual oversight compels Kant to devote much more attention to time as a form of intuition than to space. In fact so definitive is time for Kant's understanding of intuition, that he conceives of space as the sequential counting off of units of distance, a conception clearly borrowed from time.[30]

Thus Hegel emphasizes that the concept is related primarily to the identity of being, which is present as a contrary in the inherent opposition of sensible intuition. We might flesh out the point by emphasizing that intuition is related primarily to the identity of thinking in that same opposition. Thus, in opposition to Kant, Hegel identifies thought, not with subject/being/space/concept, but with predicate/thinking/time/intuition. Thus thought, for Hegel, is discursive, dialectical, speculative. Reason here will not stop short at opposition, but will press to resolve opposition in absolute identity.

Hegel professes that Kant has opened the way to solving the opposition of concept and intuition with the formulation of his question: How are synthetic judgments *a priori* possible? For, according to Hegel, they are possible through the original, absolute identity of the elements separated in judgments, namely, subject and predicate, particular and universal, sensible intuition and concept. Hegel insists that what Kant calls the *a priori* aspect of judgments is in truth the identity of these elements in reason. However, for Kant, this identity takes the form of the copula in judgments. This bare 'is', though, remains something unconscious, an unthought and unknown element. Thus, for Hegel, the judgment itself is only the prevailing appearance of difference; the sinking of reason into opposition; the unknowability of reason. Accordingly, though the Kantian treatment of judgment presupposes the absolute identity of reason, it does so only unconsciously.[31]

Hegel attempts to raise to consciousness the unconscious identity of reason in the Kantian philosophy by isolating what Kant calls the capacity of the original synthetic unity of apperception. This capacity, otherwise known as the productive imagination, functions in Kant's theory as a two-sided identity, at once that of the subject in general and that of the object. But, Hegel presses, it must not be overlooked that the productive imagination is the original unity of experience, and it is no less than the appearance of reason in the sphere of empirical consciousness:

> This power of imagination is the original two-sided identity. The identity becomes subject in general on one side, and object on the other; but originally it is both. And the imagination is nothing but Reason itself, the Idea of which was determined above. But it is only Reason as it appears in the sphere of empirical consciousness. (Ibid. p. 73)

As such the productive imagination would be the identity of concept and intuition, ego and world, intelligence and nature.[32] Thus Hegel identifies Kant's genuine contribution not to be the discovery of the categories as the absolutely finite limits of human experience. Much rather Kant should be seen to have established a foothold for the philosophy of speculative reason. But, Hegel maintains, Kant quite consciously insisted upon repressing the productive imagination and denying to understanding the capacity of intuition. He was thus left with a notion of understanding which attested to the empty formality of reason. Kant then sought for the fulfillment of reason in the sphere of practice and belief in an absolute beyond.[33]

Reason, according to Hegel, was thus made into a "dimensionless activity", as the pure concept of infinity opposed to the finite, and as a pure unity devoid of intuition. This, however, entails a contradiction, in Hegel's judgment:

> As freedom, Reason is supposed to be absolute, yet the essence of this freedom consists in being solely through an opposite. (Ibid. p. 81)

Kant's philosophy cannot survive the contradiction involved in positing freedom as absolute infinity when it is in truth conditioned by the opposition to the finite. The real failure of this system is apparent, he continues, in the claim that the absolute emptiness of such an infinity gives itself a content in practical reason, and extends that content through duty. Theoretical reason, which only has the role of regulating the manifold of understanding given to it in experience, can lay claim neither to the dignity of autonomy nor to spontaneity.

Hegel thus identifies a polemic against reason in Kant's philosophy. He points to the paralogisms and antinomies of the Transcendental Dialectic of the *Critique of Pure Reason* in substantiation of this claim. In the paralogisms, Hegel argues, Kant's sole interest is to raise the empirical ego to the level of an intellectual ego. He does not attempt to see the ego as a form of understanding which belongs to spirit. Nor does he have in mind a real, existing monad, or substance. Instead Kant presents the ego as a fixed *intellectual* unity of the infinite opposition of the finite and the infinite. To conceive of the ego in this way is, according to Hegel, to make it the absolute of finitude.[34]

In the so-called mathematical antinomies (those belonging to intuition, i.e., the first and second antinomies of the first *Critique*) Kant presents the simple negativity of reason. Here reason is fixed in reflection as the production of empirical infinity in the insurmountable contradiction of thesis and antithesis. The resolution of the mathematical antinomies is, according to Hegel, only the negative work of reason, for it involves denying the reality in-itself of both thesis and antithesis. Thus Kant suppresses the positive element of reason in these antinomies, namely, the mediation of thesis and antithesis as they are in themselves. This, Hegel points out, serves the aim of practical reason, in that it turns reason away from the infinite regress and toward the realization of its incapacity, in the name of absolute freedom.[35]

The solution of the so-called dynamical antinomies (those belonging to understanding, i.e., the third and the fourth antinomies of the first *Critique*) marks, in Hegel's judgment, a genuine advance. For this discovers the absolute dualism of Kant's philosophy. The oppositions of freedom and nature, and of an intelligible and a sensible world, are made absolute. This serves, despite Kant's intention, to posit their absolute identity in pure form.[36]

Hegel notes that the solution to the dynamical antinomies is not merely thought, but categorially posited in Kant's treatment of speculative theology, especially with regard to the ontological proof for the existence of God. Unfortunately, Hegel remarks, Kant deals with this proof in a lesser form, in which existence is taken to be a characteristic of God (rather than as God's essence), and so he fails to expose the full positivity of the opposition of thinking and being.

After having proceeded through the promise and shortcomings of Kant's theoretical and practical philosophies of reason, Hegel focuses upon the important critique of judgment. For here, he avers, we find the most interesting element of Kantian philosophy: a region which stands between the empirical manifold and the absolute, abstract unity (of understanding), but which is nevertheless not a region of knowledge.

In the reflective faculty of judgment Kant discovers the middle term between the concept of nature and the concept of freedom. This region remains unsurpassed both by the theoretical and the practical philosophies of Kant, as it comprises the absolute judgment of subject and predicate. And, though Kant deals with the reality of reason here in a formal manner, Hegel identifies this as the sole true appearance of reason. For in this region are conjoined conscious intuition (in beauty) and unconscious intuition (in the organization of nature).[37]

Hegel's analysis of Kant's *Critique of Judgement* focuses upon the antinomy of taste: on one hand it is thought that there is no accounting for taste, and on the other that there is ample room for disagreement in matters of taste. The basis of this antinomy, for Kant, is that judgments of taste are made without the use of a concept, and yet are criticized by means of a concept. The solution to this antinomy Kant presents is to recognize that the concept of taste in question is indeterminate. Thus it is true that judgments of taste involve no determinate concept by which they are formulated. It is also true that such judgments can be quarreled over on the basis of an indeterminate concept of taste. This indeterminate concept Kant calls the super-sensible which underlies both the object and the subject judging it in its phenomenal appearance.[38]

Hegel finds this a specious treatment of the matter. Kant, he remarks, claims that the undetermined idea of the super-sensible in us cannot be made further conceptual. But, Hegel contends, Kant has already presented this concept in the identity of the concept of nature and of freedom. Kant avers that an aesthetic idea cannot be knowable, because it is an intuition of the productive imagination to which no concept is adequate. He likewise asserts that an idea of reason cannot be knowable, because it includes a concept of the super-sensible to which an intuition is never adequate. However, Hegel maintains that the aesthetic idea has its exposition in the idea of reason; that the idea of reason has its exposition in beauty.[39]

Hegel explains this oversight of Kant by comparing the antinomy of taste to the mathematical antinomies of the first *Critique*. In both cases the idea of reason is posited at once as something purely sensible and as super-sensible. Thus the antinomy of taste, as those of the world and the thing, is resolved in Kant by taking the super-sensible in a negative (regulative) sense.[40] Judgments of taste, according to Kant, are capable of being disputed only on the basis of an unknown. Hegel thus notes that for Kant the super-sensible is beyond knowledge: neither is it intuited in the beautiful; nor is it the identity of freedom and nature; least of all is it the ground of the perennial opposition of the sensible and the super-sensible.[41] For Hegel, manifestly it is all of these.[42]

Kant's treatment of the objective side of the matter (the unconscious intuition of the reality of reason, or organic nature) in the critique of teleological judgment comes closer, in Hegel's view, to the idea of reason. Here Kant refers to an intuitive understanding and the consequent unity of actuality and possibility. Kant claims that we are compelled toward this idea, and yet he finally and decisively distributes understanding to concepts, and sensible intuition to objects. Thus, Hegel concludes, the idea though necessary is problematic. But the matter has already gone too far:

> Yet he himself thinks an intuitive intellect and is led to it as an absolutely necessary Idea....He himself shows that his cognitive faculty is aware not only of the appearance and of the separation of the possible and the actual in it, but also of Reason and the In-itself. Kant has here before him both the Idea of a Reason in which possibility and actuality are absolutely identical and its appearance as cognitive faculty wherein they are separated. (Ibid. p. 89)

And yet, Hegel charges, Kant disdains to think necessity, reason, and an intuitive spontaneity, and chooses instead for mere appearance.

Hegel is adamant that Kant knows it is possible for the mechanism of nature and teleological technism to exist in and of themselves in an original, absolute identity. This, we might add, is shown in Kant's presentation of the antinomy of teleology. For here he argues that we must judge products of material nature as all arising from mechanical laws, and yet some as arising, not from mechanical laws, but from final causes.[43] Despite this, Hegel points out, Kant takes reason, as the higher principle of nature (encompassing final causes), to be transcendent. Thus Kant qualifies: for *human* reason the identity of nature and reason is not a possibility.[44]

Kant notwithstanding, Hegel avers, in beauty we have an intuition which is not of the sensible, and so too a form of knowledge beyond that of appearance. Hegel asserts, Kant has, in full consciousness of this possibility, destroyed the highest idea, and raised finite knowledge above it.[45] In so doing Kant has left us with the mere faith in what Hegel characterizes as an "absolute unthought, unknown, inconceivable beyond."[46]

Hegel summarizes his criticism thusly: If we strip the practical faith of Kantian philosophy, namely, faith in God, of the unphilosophical and popular clothes in which it is dressed, we have nothing but the idea that reason should have absolute reality; so that in this idea all opposition between freedom and necessity is transcended; so that infinite thinking is absolute reality, or the absolute identity of thinking and being. But this idea is none other than that known to true philosophy as the first and only, namely, the ontological proof of the existence of God.[47] The speculative element of this idea is of course decanted by Kant in human form, so that morality and happiness are harmonized in the notion of the highest good of the world, so that this thought of heaven would thus be realized. Hegel's response is the following, "... --something as wretched as this morality and this happiness the highest good!" (Ibid. p. 94f.)

B. Jacobi.

Hegel's criticism of Jacobi follows directly from the preceding analysis of Kant. For, whereas Kant failed in the end to admit the full objectivity of the Absolute in reason, Jacobi presents the Absolute as pure subjectivity. Thus Kant's philosophy here comes to represent at least the possibility of speculative knowledge, while Jacobi is portrayed as opposing that possibility in his every move. Jacobi's philosophy rejects even the formal objectivity of the Absolute found in Kant's concepts of the understanding.

Yet in Jacobi's polemic against the Kantian philosophy, Hegel sees a radicalizing of subjectivity itself which supersedes any sense of subjectivity found in Kant. Jacobi, then, marks a crucial stage in the development of reason toward the absolute opposition between subjectivity and objectivity. And this opposition provides an avenue for grasping the Absolute through genuinely speculative knowledge.

According to Hegel the philosophies of Kant and Jacobi share the common ground of absolute finitude. Finitude and subjectivity have the objective form of the concept in Kant's philosophy. In Jacobi's, however, finitude and subjectivity are fashioned as individuality.[48] Thus, while Kant and Jacobi share the common ground of finitude, they nevertheless are opposed to one another with regard to the subjectivity of knowledge.

Because Jacobi developed a philosophy diametrically opposed to that of Kant, his position exposes a possibility overlooked in the Kantian theory, namely, that of grasping the genuine beauty of experience. And, this, as we saw in the preceding section, is precisely that possibility conclusively obviated by the Kantian philosophy.

Hegel's presentation begins with an analysis of the subjectivization of knowledge in Jacobi's philosophy. First Jacobi abstracts the form of knowledge and presents it in its purity. Hegel describes this formal knowledge as an "identity of the understanding" which is supposed to receive its content and thus its reality from the empirical sphere. The empirical here, Hegel notes, represents the sole aspect of objectivity to be found in Jacobi's theory of knowledge. Without this Jacobi's conception of knowledge is purely formal, concerning itself only with the principle of identity.[49]

The formal identity of knowledge in Jacobi amounts to the capacity of recognizing relations. The principle of identity means: whatever it is, it is just that (*quidquid est, illud est*). Proceeding by way of this principle, knowledge can only discover varying degrees of similarity between one object and another. And, because such knowledge depends upon comparison and approximation, it can never be complete and certain. The sole true basis of certainty, according to Jacobi, is "faith", and rational knowledge must rely upon this for its own certainty. For in the end knowledge is itself only an approximation of the certainty proper to faith.[50]

Hegel's analysis shows that Jacobi has given a far more subjective account of the unity of knowledge than Kant. Kant provides knowledge with the objective unity of the pure concepts of understanding, or the categories. Jacobi reduces this unity to a thoroughgoing subjectivity. For he replaces the categories with the table of judgments, and then discards everything from the table of judgments, save the identical judgment. Claiming this as the only form of apodeictic knowledge, Jacobi then makes even the identical judgment dependent upon a preceding certainty of faith. Thus knowledge is reduced to the principle of identity, and identity is seen to rest upon faith.

According to Hegel, however, the principle of identity has a necessary counterpart in Jacobi's philosophy. That counterpart is the principle of sufficient reason,[51] and here, as with the principle of identity, it is clear that Jacobi works a subjectivizing influence upon the theory of knowledge.

The laying down of the principle of sufficient reason bears witness, in Hegel's opinion, to the striving of past philosophical development toward reason. Hegel suggests, however, that this principle has been variously taken up as an expression of reason or of reflection. In the case of Jacobi, he remarks, it is clear that the principle of sufficient reason is taken in the latter way. For Jacobi distinguishes the logical aspect of this principle from its causal aspect. Thus, in his philosophy, the principle of sufficient reason has sometimes to do with the relation of ground and proposition, and at others with the relation of cause and effect.[52]

Hegel notes that in Jacobi the principle of sufficient reason is tied to the age-old problem of the part and the whole. Thus Jacobi at least begins his treatment of this principle with an important finding of reason:

> *totum parte prius esse necesse est* [the whole is necessarily prior to the part] .... In other words, the single part only gets determined in the whole. It has its reality only in the absolute identity which, insofar as discernibles are posited in it, is absolute totality. (Ibid. p. 99)

However Jacobi takes the statement of reason (that the whole is necessarily prior to the part) in two ways. In one sense (apparently as logical relation) it means: the identical is the self-same (*idem est idem*). In another sense (presumably as causal relation) it means something else.[53] According to Hegel, Jacobi struggles to keep these two senses of the statement separate. In its logical aspect Jacobi takes the principle of sufficient reason as the principle of pure contradiction.[54] Apparently what Hegel means is that Jacobi conceives of the principle of sufficient reason along the lines of the principle of non-contradiction: A is A and not something else. Thus the ground, A, is not the consequence, B, and so the consequence is the contradiction of the ground. Accordingly, Hegel notes, for Jacobi the principle of sufficient reason would be an abstract unity, save that the empirical is necessarily added to it to account for the difference of ground and consequence. On the other hand, Jacobi takes the principle of sufficient reason to represent a causal relation. Here the heterogenous element of the empirical (the effect) is said to be added to the identity of the concept (the cause), and so the principle of sufficient reason is claimed as a concept of experience (rather than as an expression of reason).

Generally, what is wrong with Jacobi's treatment of the principle of sufficient reason, in Hegel's judgment, is that his notion of totality is one which lacks the parts. Consequently Jacobi must search about for them in the realm of the empirical, and add them to the whole. Thus the whole as such lacks the objective elements of succession and becoming, and so is taken to be subjective in kind.

The principle of sufficient reason is the necessary counterpart to the principle of identity in Jacobi's philosophy, because the former is taken up in the form of the principle of contradiction. Thus the principle of identity, A is A, is paired with the principle of sufficient reason, A is A and not B. The implication Hegel draws out of this is that, in Jacobi's philosophy, the principle of identity presupposes the principle of sufficient reason: "A is A" means "A is not B". Thus, not only the principle of sufficient reason, but also that of identity presupposes the supervention of the empirical in order to account for the difference between A and everything else. To construe these principles in this fashion, Hegel avers, is to present them as thoroughly subjective, abstract, and empty formalities of knowledge.

The crucial item that arises from out of Hegel's analysis of the principles of identity and sufficient reason in Jacobi is the relation of time and eternity. For, in attempting to arrive at a proper conception of the Absolute, it must be determined how the Absolute is related both to time and to eternity.

In the first *Critique* Kant provides an account of the relation of the categories to the sensible manifold. Though this account takes various forms,[55] generally it attempts to establish time as the relation obtaining between the categories and sense data. Thus the relations expressed in the concept of cause or succession, in Kant, are thought to be mediated by time. As conditioned by time, all such relations between the categories and the sensible manifold necessarily belong to the sphere of appearance.

Jacobi essayed a deduction that was to surpass that of Kant. Hegel scrutinizes this attempt. Jacobi, he notes, posits succession as prior to time. Time, Jacobi argues, is the representation of succession. But prior even to succession is the fundamental relation of action and reaction arising out of a thing that senses and the thing sensed: the action of touching something is met by the reaction of impenetrability.[56] Thus, contrary to Kant, Jacobi would have it that the mediation of concepts and sensation occurs in the consciousness of action and reaction, rather than in time. And, since this consciousness is prior to time, Jacobi claims that the fundamental relation of action and reaction is attributable, not to mere appearances, but to things as they are in themselves.[57]

In Hegel's judgment, all Jacobi has accomplished in this deduction is to render absolute what in Kant is appearance. For underlying all of Jacobi's notions is the simple presupposition of a community of single things. And it is the sphere of such finite empirical objects that is to provide human consciousness with absolute objectivity.[58] But, in Hegel's opinion, to restrict philosophy to the sphere of the finite is to abandon it. It is the task of philosophy to think the Absolute, to grasp the finite together with the infinite, the temporal together with the eternal.[59] But the polarized philosophy of reflection always conceives things asymmetrically. Hegel sums up the matter as follows:

> This is the eternal dilemma of reflection: if philosophy recognizes a transition from the eternal to the temporal, it can easily be shown that philosophy posits the temporal in the eternal itself and therefore makes the eternal temporal. On the other hand, if philosophy does not recognize this transition, if it posits that for intuitive cognition totality is an absolute *simul*, an absolute together, so that the different [i.e., the manifold of differentiated particulars] does not exist in the form of [spatial] parts and temporality, then philosophy is deficient, for it is supposed to have the temporal, the determinate, and the single before it and explain that also. (Ibid. p. 127)

It is the latter option which Jacobi chooses, according to Hegel, claiming that philosophy represents a mere formal grasp of the absolute *simul*, or the eternal, to which must be added the temporal.[60] Thus he posits the absoluteness of the finite (the temporal), and attempts to account for its relation to the absoluteness of the subjectivity of knowledge (the eternal).

For Jacobi, the relation of the temporal to the eternal is called faith. This faith, Hegel remarks, has two sides. On one hand, it represents the non-conceptual knowledge of particulars, or the immediate grasp of the temporal upon which all knowledge is based.[61] On the other hand, faith has as its object the eternal. This form of faith is also non-conceptual, for it sees in cognition only something formal and subjective.[62]

The type of faith embraced by Jacobi, according to Hegel, has the effect of limiting faith itself to the naive grasp of the temporal, and thus also of denying all knowledge of the eternal. But when faith is introduced to philosophy, as in Jacobi, it is turned into a flight from the temporal and a suspension of the eternal. For faith in the immediate certainty of the temporal is taken by philosophy to be faith in the eternal. The finitude of temporality is nullified, and the subjectivity of eternity is cancelled: every finite thing is thought to present itself under an eternal shape. For example, one's finite actions and perceptions alternate with divine worship, so that one's own conduct is thought to express the eternal. But, Hegel argues, this too is subjective, for it is nothing more than the ethical beauty of the individual. Reflection upon the subjectivity of this faith under the name of philosophy serves only to pollute it by preserving the element of subjectivity in it, even as a nullity.[63]

Jacobi's treatment of faith in his philosophy is thus, according to Hegel, preoccupied with the personality and fixated upon eternal self-contemplation.[64] The problem of faith and reflection here involved is summed up in the following passage:

> Thus, in Jacobi Protestant subjectivity seems to return out of the Kantian conceptual form to its true shape, to a subjective beauty of feeling (*Empfindung*) and to a lyrical yearning for heaven. But faith and individual beauty now have an essential ingredient of reflection and of consciousness of this subjective beauty, and are thus cast out of that state of innocence and unreflectedness which alone makes them capable of being beautiful, devout and religious. (Ibid. p. 147)

Hegel concludes that, directly contrary to Kant's insistence upon the objectivity and infinity of the concept, Jacobi makes a principle out of finitude as empirical contingency and subjective consciousness. Thus common to both is the absolute antithesis between finite, natural knowledge and the infinite, supernatural supersensuous. Accordingly, for both, the Absolute remains beyond cognitive reason, an object of mere faith and feeling. Likewise, in both philosophies the speculative idea emerges for a time, only to be sundered in the end. In Kant's philosophy this idea is present in the deduction of the categories, but only as the unity of the understanding itself or as the possible thought which can never become actual. In Jacobi, on the other hand, the speculative idea is present in personality, though only as subjective individuality.[65] What is lacking in both, therefore, is the intellectual intuition, i.e., the idea, which grasps the intelligible and the sensible, the eternal and the temporal, under the form of the Absolute.

In Hegel's judgment, Jacobi must be ranked below Kant, as regards knowledge. Kant at least presents the objectivity of knowledge in a form that can be seen to suggest the role of reason. Jacobi, however, denies reason any significant place in his philosophy. But, as regards faith, clearly Jacobi marks an improvement upon Kant. For Kant, faith remains nothing more than a hypothesis for understanding and a postulate for moral conduct. In Jacobi, on the other hand, faith has initially at least the proper form of the subjective beauty of the individual. The positive aspect of Jacobi's philosophy, according to Hegel, is that it comes close in principle to the truth of Protestantism. The individual and the particular are placed above the concept, and so subjective vivacity is underscored. Consciousness of the divine is conceived as something inward which abides by its inwardness. And though this yearning for the Absolute cannot be realized, its object is in truth the eternal.[66] The negative side of this, in Hegel's opinion, is this: faith in the eternal alone has a polemical character which inevitably reflects back into subjectivity. Being thus subjective, moreover, this faith has the aspect of certitude. Consequently it turns toward the temporal and actual, so that the witness of the senses is made to serve as the revelation of truth, and feeling and instinct are taken to comprise the rule of conduct. But such certitude, Hegel remarks, can do nothing to assuage the grief of religious yearning.[67]

Hegel's analysis shows that Jacobi's philosophy presents a conception of faith true to the grief and yearning of Prostestantism. But it also points out that the reconciliation of this grief and yearning cannot be found in certitude arising out of the temporal and actual, as Jacobi professes. For the finite, according to Hegel, is nothing else than the reflective consciousness of grief and yearning itself.[68]

C. Fichte.

Hegel's critical remarks on Fichte's philosophy once more address the matter of subjectivity. Knowledge in Fichte, as in Kant and Jacobi, is merely formal. Accordingly, Hegel avers, the knowing subject is always distanced from the proper object of knowledge, namely, the Absolute. Thus faith in an absolute Beyond is introduced in the attempt to grasp what for cognition remains unattainable. The subjectivity of this philosophy, even when decked out in the objectifying formulas of ethical action, remains a stumbling block to reason, and so must be exposed, corrected, and ultimately superseded.

Hegel rehearses the relation between the philosophies of Kant, Jacobi, and Fichte in the opening passages of this section. Kant, he reminds, places thinking first in his system, as the universal form of the objective, or the infinite. In absolute opposition to this we find being, the particular, or the finite. The opposition between thinking and being is located in the knowing subject, but it remains below the level of consciousness. Therefore the absolute identity in which thinking and being are one never emerges in the Kantian philosophy, except as mere surmise, or faith. Jacobi, on the other hand, places the consciousness of this antithesis first in his philosophy. And by transposing the opposition from the realm of cognition to that of faith, this philosophy gives the appearance of having resolved the antithesis between thinking and being. In truth it has only provided a discursive account of the yearning and grief of Protestant piety. Finally, in the philosophy of Fichte the subjective yearning of Jacobi is provided a Kantian veneer of objectivity. The union of the subject with living individuality, i.e., personality, is presented in an objective form. This subjectivity of yearning is made into the culmination of Fichte's system. Hegel formulates it thus: I *ought* also to be not-I.[69]

Hegel's analysis of Fichte's philosophy thus focuses upon the role of the *ought* (*Sollen*) as the middle term between thinking and being. According to the ethics of Kant, the move from theoretical philosophy to practical philosophy is made possible by the truth that *ought* implies *can*. That is, given a sense of obligation (expressed here in the word, ought), one says that this obligation can be fulfilled, in principle. Else the moral sense would be an absurd superfluity to the intractable course of nature. Thus obligation presupposes the possibility of fulfillment, or as Kant puts it: ought implies can.

Fichte picks up on Kant's formula, and applies it directly to the ego: I ought to be not-I. The gist of Fichte's adaptation of the formula is that the self encounters its own perceptions. These perceptions are collectively called the not-I. However, the I on its own knows itself to be radically incomplete, and so it strives to complete itself by becoming what it is not, namely, the not-I. The self ought to become its perceptions.

Hegel maintains, against Kant and Fichte, that, though ought implies can, can in no way implies is. Indeed it would seem that, for Hegel, ought precludes is. For, in one sense of the word, when I say, for example, that I *ought* to be diligent, manifestly I *am not*. In another sense, however, it might be said, that I *ought* to be a student of philosophy, when in fact I *am*. What is meant here is: I am a student of philosophy, and it is well. Hegel takes the 'ought' of Kant and Fichte, however, in the former sense. This obligation implies, in his account, not only that the I is not the not-I, but that it never can be so.[70] A closer look at his analysis of Fichte will make as much clear.

Hegel notes that Fichte's system comprises three elements. The first is represented by positing, thinking, and infinity, the second by opposition, being, and finitude. The third is the relation of the first two, and is sub-divided into a) positive knowledge, as the relation of thinking to being and b) the absolute identity of thinking and being.[71] Hegel's analysis of this triplicity reveals the shortcomings of Fichte's system. The first two elements in question make up the basic opposition between thinking and being. The first element itself is represented in the equation: I=I. This is the formal unity of knowledge, the infinite, which stands opposed to the finite. The second element is the necessary correlate to the first, and is expressed: not-I. Underivable from the I, this element is the finite which opposes the infinite. The third element combines the first two elements through the causal nexus, on one hand, and through faith, on the other.[72]

According to Hegel, the relating of thinking and being through the principle of causation bears a characteristic incompleteness. The subject relates itself to its object, as I to not-I, either through the free causality of moral action or the natural causality of perception. However, in either case, it is the incompleteness of the I that compels it to seek to think. Because the I does not perceive or intuit things, but rather only its own perceptions and intuitions, its first certainty is the pure activity of empty knowing: "...there is strictly nothing but pure knowing, and pure intuiting, and sensing: Ego=Ego" (Ibid., p. 156). This incompleteness of the absolute principle of self-consciousness in Fichte's philosophy necessitates a deduction of the objective world. The first principle, I=I, in being incomplete, has within it the immediate necessity of self-fulfillment. It must go out of itself to something else, and from there to the infinity of the empirical world. The necessity of this deduction lies in the fact that the I is a mere part which must seek its completion in the whole. Thus the objective world comes on the scene as the completion of the I.[73]

Hegel describes this deduction as an elaborate tautology. Beginning with the certainty and truth of pure knowing, the I proceeds to pick up one intuition or perception after the other. It strings this series of parts together, and claims the whole as the world. But, Hegel remarks, this is only to pick up again what was previously abstracted from in the act of pure knowing.[74] In other words, says Hegel, this deduction amounts to nothing more than positing again what has already been negated. As regards the causality of nature, this involves first abstracting from the world of sense, and then positing that world as a condition of self-consciousness.[75] In the sphere of free causality, on the other hand, the objective world in which ethical actions transpire is abstracted from, and then posited again as being.

According to Hegel, Fichte's deduction of the world does not truly complete the I. For the I, though it is a part in need of the whole, does not know itself to be a part. Instead it takes itself as an empty whole which must be filled with the serial parts of the empirical, or objective world. But, since there is no intuition of the whole to which the I could relate itself as a part, it can never complete itself, not even through an infinity of piecemeal additions.[76]

Because of the emptiness of knowing in Fichte, Hegel maintains, the I is nothing more than a formal unity. The first principle of Fichte's system, I=I, means to Hegel: I=Nothing. Moreover, the second principle of the system, not-I, becomes, in Hegel's reading: ought. The not-I is the principle which states that the I ought to be. Thus the third principle of the system states, on one hand, that nothing (I) causes what ought (not-I) to be, and on the other, that nothing and what ought are absolutely identical in faith. Thus thinking and being ought to be coincident, and in faith they are, as yearning.[77] However the coincidence of thinking and being remains, according to Hegel, a mere ideal even in faith. For in Fichte's conception of the realm of faith, what ought to be (the not-I) is construed as the moral order of the world, and yet this too remains outside the I. The moral order attains reality, in Fichte's philosophy, only in an infinite process. And, if this process were ever to become complete, the I would become the not-I; the I would cease to be as I:

> In Fichte too, the moral world order that exists in things simply cannot become for the Ego what they ought to be, precisely because, if they did, the non-Ego would cease to be and become Ego. (Ibid. p. 170)

The consequence of Fichte's philosophy for faith, according to Hegel, is that faith must be thought of as the never-ending yearning of the I for its completion in the not-I. But the presupposition of this thought is just that principle which guides Jacobi's philosophy: *Either* God exists and exists *outside* me, a living being subsisting apart; or *else* I am God. *There is no third way.*[78] And, since the I cannot become the Absolute, for Fichte, the only possibility left is that God remains unattainable, removed to the Beyond of faith.

D. Conclusion.

In the conclusion to the article on faith and knowledge Hegel's anticipation is high:

> This metaphysic of subjectivity has run through the complete cycle of its forms in the philosophies of Kant, Jacobi, and Fichte ....The

metaphysic of subjectivity has, therefore, completely set forth [the intrinsic stages of] the formative process of culture; for this formative process consists in establishing as absolute each of the [two] single dimensions [of being and thought, object and subject, etc.] of the totality and elaborating each of them into a system. The metaphysic of subjectivity has brought this cultural process to its end. Therewith the external possibility directly arises that the true philosophy should emerge out of this [completed] culture, nullify the absoluteness of its finitudes and present itself all at once as perfected appearance, with all its riches subjected to the totality. (Ibid. p. 189)

The absolute opposition between the finite and the infinite is exposed in the philosophy of reflection. Hegel thus attempts to prove the claim that the principle of the North and of Protestantism --the absolute subjectivity of yearning for an otherworldly and unattainable God-- has reached a crisis in the culture of the age. That this crisis emerged despite the express intentions of the leading minds of the Enlightenment demonstrates all the more convincingly to Hegel that the event is one of fate.

In failing to press beyond the limitations of understanding, the Enlightenment accepted the lot of eudaemonism, forgoing the possibility of eternal happiness. The philosophy of reflection refused to think God, and settled instead for earthly satisfaction. And yet, Hegel avers, the philosophy of the empty infinite is all the closer to the true speculative philosophy, because it conceives of the infinite as indifference.[79] And indifference is the proper relation of the finite and the infinite. The fatefulness of this conception is expressed epigrammatically in the saying that God is dead.

Hegel charges that the empty infinity of the philosophy of reflection must be seen to give a philosophical existence to the feeling that God is dead;[80] that the thought of the Enlightenment is finally nothing but an account of knowledge as the formal activity of the subject; that all strictly conceptual thought is without an object; that thinking under the aegis of the understanding precludes being; that to think God is not to know that God exists--this must be seen as the intellectual basis of the infinite pain which accompanies the feeling that God is dead. To see this is, according to Hegel, to grasp that the highest form of philosophizing is, not the concept, but much rather the idea. To see that the philosophy of the understanding justifies the feeling that God is dead is to realize that the speculative philosophy of the idea can transform the grief of the Enlightenment. It is to see that the yearning for an already dead God presupposes the highest idea, namely, that to think God is to know that he exists, even in death. All that remains to be seen is how Hegel purports to think God. But this is no easy task. Indeed Hegel attempts nothing along these lines in the present article.

Yet Hegel's claim that the philosophy of reflection furnishes the death of God with its conceptual form, raises again the issue of criticism and the underlying problem of interpretation. Kant, Jacobi, and Fichte each avowed belief in God. Kant was admittedly ordered to stop publishing on the subject of theology because of his controversial views, but he defended his genuine belief in God.[81] Fichte in his turn lost his post under suspicion of atheism arising from his system of philosophy, and yet he never tired of disclaiming the truth of the allegation.[82] Jacobi, though he suggested he was a pagan in his thinking, confessed that in his heart he was a Christian.[83] Indeed no thinker of the day could be oblivious to the repressive policies of the new Weimar government and its promise to punish all who strayed from the teachings of Biblical doctrine. These, then, were not superficial and idle insinuations Hegel was making. In identifying these three thinkers, not only as the leading, but as the necessary mouthpieces of the saying that God is dead he was leaving them and himself open to controversy. And, it must not be overlooked that these thinkers never referred to such a thought as the death of God in their own writings. Was Hegel guilty of putting dangerous words in their mouths?

In answering this question it should first be noted that, though Hegel employs the phrase "God Himself is dead", these words are on his admission not his own. Even without the references to Pascal and Lutheranism (from which the words actually stem) it is clear that Hegel is not offering these words as his own. They are set off in the text by punctuation which suggests that they belong to someone else. Secondly, Hegel never shied in his critical articles from saying more about an author's words than that author himself might have said. But, if we accept Hegel's hermeneutical concept of criticism as the attempt to discover in the individual words of an author the universal truth of philosophy, we cannot at the same time accuse him of claiming those words for any given author, himself included. Thus, with regard to the death of God, Hegel is here neither absolving himself from any responsibility for these words by placing them in the mouth of another, nor is he accepting full responsibility for them as a individual author. Rather his responsibility is that of a critic with a view to why criticism is worth taking a certain risk. He would, it seems, take full responsibility for seeing in the philosophy of the Enlightenment that the words "God Himself is dead" cannot help but come to speech, but, it also seems, only so long as those words are justified by the idea of philosophy. This is an important point, for Hegel would surely be guilty of hypocrisy, if he expected others to share his responsibility, except by way of partaking in the idea of philosophy emergent in the sources and content of the *Critical Journal of Philosophy*. For he never tired of decrying the urge of philosophers to gain approval for an idea by broad or even universal consent of their peers.

If we are to take Hegel at his best, we must conclude that he wrote these words in solitude, for himself. The saying that God is dead is uttered in a *tete a tete* between Hegel and the idea of philosophy, and the alienation of such a thought is only the more apparent when this conversation is made public for all to see.

Yet, lest the element of solitude overshadow Hegel's utterance and render it nothing but a private confession, it should be noted that the death of God epitomizes what Hegel referred to as an event of the world-spirit. His critical reading of philosophy, we must assume, was not to be taken as a local and temporary event in the first years of Germany's 19th century, any more than the philosophy of the Enlightenment which he criticized was to be so taken. The saying that God is dead is as much a part of the fate of philosophy as are the systems which gave rise to it. The point is to realize that thinking, critical and philosophical alike, is an affair of fate. And, if that fate entails the feeling that God is dead, its truth and reality cannot be denied to thought. The harshness of the saying must be known to any who would dare to philosophize, for to philosophize is learn to die, even if it be God who must die.

Finally, it might be added that in uttering the saying that God has died Hegel has accepted the fate of leaving reading behind for writing. He has given up criticism for philosophy. This point need not be argued on the basis of the doubtful state of Hegel's so-called system at the time of his publishing *Glauben und Wissen*. The resolve to become a philosopher need not be supported by the existence of sketches of a system either immediately before or after the decision. The evidence that Hegel was becoming a philosophy is ample in the text itself. The lucidity of style and cogency of the article on faith and knowledge is witness to a new calling. None of the other articles of the journal portray such clearness of thought and expression. It is as though Hegel wrote this article with a conviction and ease unknown to the other pieces, because this and not those was his watershed. And should we not expect a change in one who has uttered such a thought?

That Hegel had now begun to write as a philosopher is also supported by the content of the other journal articles. The introductory article outlined the concept of criticism to be employed in the service of the idea of philosophy. The next two articles by Hegel, on common sense and scepticism, are impatient pieces, struggling all the while to bolt ahead to the piece on the reflection-philosophy. Enough allusions to reflection-philosophy are made in the two previous articles to indicate that the *intentio* of Hegel's project would lead him to the utterance of the death of God. This sense of anticipation is communicated to the reader, who intuits early on that the subject of the criticisms of common sense and scepticism is indeed something beyond positivistic empiricism and the history of scepticism. When one finally makes it to the article on faith and knowledge, it becomes clear from the first sentence that Hegel was all the while making his way toward the philosophy of reflection and its dire consequence. And, surely the meaning of that consequence would be incomprehensible to one who had not read the previous articles. For the opposition between the empirical and the conceptual, between being and thinking, which is so much attended in *Glauben und Wissen* is fully intelligible only when it is seen that these have their respective roots in common sense and scepticism. At once the reader sees the force of the opposition throughout the history of philosophy which finally climaxes in the conflict of the eudaemonist empiricism of practical philosophy and the stoic scepticism of theoretical philosophy. By depicting these as the cultural bedfellows of the Enlightenment, Hegel shows us the dire straits of the time: thought cannot truly think itself. No wonder philosophy opts out of the situation by fleeing into pietism. The flight of Enlightenment philosophy both supports and seeks support from a form of religion based in the feeling that God is unthinkable, save as dead. Yet to think the death of God is to recognize in modernity a new age and time, a new fate which, because it is intuited in advance, is no longer fate, but rather has become destiny. That Hegel made this his destiny is attested by the last of Hegel's journal articles, to which we now turn.

ENDNOTES

[1]Cerf and Harris, *Faith and Knowledge*, p. 190f. All the material in the parentheses and the brackets is that of the translators.
[2]Faith, p. 62.
[3]SW Vol. 1, p. 286.
[4]Ibid. p. 288.
[5]Ibid. p. 281.
[6]Ibid. p. 279.
[7]Ibid. p. 279f.
[8]Ibid. p. 281.
[9]Ibid. p. 282.
[10]Ibid. p. 282f.
[11]This may well be because Hegel recognized that this was in his day already a failed ideal. See Sunlight, pp. 353-55 on this topic.
[12]SW Vol. 1, p. 283f.
[13]Ibid. p. 284.
[14]Ibid. p. 285f.
[15]Ibid. p. 286.
[16]This was, of course, the point of Hegel's article on scepticism considered above.
[17]Ibid. p. 291.

[18]I have provided the material in brackets for context.

[19]Ibid. p. 293.

[20]CPR p. 276.

[21]SW Vol. 1, p. 295.

[22]CPR p. 93.

[23] It must be noted that Hegel, following Kant, refers here solely to sensible, not intellectual, intuition. Kant distinguished between sensible (or derivative) and intellectual (or original intuition), and maintained that humans are capable only of the former. See, for example, CPR p. 90. Hegel's conception of intellectual intuition and its role in reason comes into play in what follows, and will be dealt with in that place.

[24]SW Vol 1, p. 297f.

[25]Kant was of two minds on this subject. In his Transcendental Aesthetic he argues that space and time are the sole forms of sensible intuition because only they are presupposed by experience. All other concepts of sensibility, e.g., motion and alteration, are derived from experience (CPR p. 81f). In the Transcendental Logic, however, Kant avers that no explanation can be given of why space and time are the only forms of sensible intuition (CPR p. 161). Hegel's advance upon Kant here is that he proffers reason as the the identity of space and time presupposed by all empirical knowledge.

[26]Kant's definition of intellectual intuition is that mode of representation which would give the existence of its object in representing the object. Intellectual intuition, he maintains, would obtain only for a being that is not finite, namely, the primordial being. See CPR p. 90. But contrast CPR p. 268 where Kant maintains that we cannot even conceive of the possibility of intellectual intuition. In any case, Kant would surely reject my examples as specious, for he would not entertain the idea of the existence of language or dream.

[27]See CPR p. 93.

[28]Cerf and Harris add an enlightening footnote in their translation of the passage under consideration:

> "This formula says that the judgment is the second 'power' (A^2) of productive imagination, the first 'power' being sensuous intuition ($A = B$). In its appearance as judgment the intellect is the reflective awareness of the identity of Subject and Predicate in their difference. Hegel's present paradigm of judgment is the subsumption of a particular under a universal (cf. above p. 69). As he takes the particulars to have the form of being and the universals to have the form of thought, he can now say that the judgment is the reflective awareness of the identity of being and thought in their difference. The next step would lead from particular beings to objects and from concepts to the the subject. So we get judgments as the reflective awareness of the identity of object and subject in their difference." (Faith, p. 71)

Though the translators speak here in terms of judgment, rather than concept, the point remains the same. Whether judgment or concept, the understanding represents only the subjective identity of intuition and concept, because it is relatively identical with the manifold of sensible, derivative intuition.

[29]That the subject is grouped with being and space is evident from Hegel's consideration of the synthetic judgment *a priori* examined above.

[30]Kant indeed claims the opposite. He maintains that the intuition of time is expressible in terms of the relations of outer appearances, namely space (CPR p. 77). However, on the other hand, he describes space as an extension *ad infinitum*, which suggests the progression of time

(CPR p. 204).

[31] SW Vol. 1, p. 300.

[32] Hegel elaborates upon these identifications on page 308f. of the present article.

[33] See ibid. p. 309f.

[34] See ibid. p. 312.

[35] Ibid. p. 313.

[36] See ibid. p. 313f.

[37] See ibid. p. 315.

[38] See *Critique of Judgement*, trans. J.H. Bernard (New York: Hafner Press, 1951), pp. 183-187.

[39] See SW Vol. 1, p. 316.

[40] See ibid. p. 317.

[41] Ibid.

[42] Ibid. p. 317.

[43] See *Critique of Judgement*, pp. 233ff.

[44] See SW Vol. 1, pp. 319ff.

[45] See ibid. p. 321f.

[46] See ibid. p. 324.

[47] Ibid.

[48] Ibid. p. 328.

[49] In quoting Jacobi Hegel writes "*Satz des Widerspruchs*" instead of "*Satz der Identität*", as found in Jacobi's text. See, *Faith and Knowledge*, p. 97, footnote 2. For the philosophical connection between these two principles upon which Hegel's "slip" is based see Heidegger's, *The Metaphysical Foundations of Logic*, trans. Michael Heim (Bloomington: Indiana University Press, 1984) p. 52f. Heidegger notes that the principle of identity is reducible to the principle of non-contradiction.

[50] See SW Vol. 1, p. 328f.

[51] The principle of sufficient reason is most often given in the form: nothing is without reason (*nihil est sine ratione*).

[52] See ibid. p. 330.

[53] Hegel's analysis is here very terse and requires some elaboration. The notion that the whole is necessarily prior to the part may be taken logically to mean that the predicate of an affirmative judgment is a part, taken in its identity with the whole represented in the subject. Thus, for example, the proposition, Socrates is a man, expresses the logical identity of the part (man) and the whole (Socrates's essence). On the other hand, the notion that the whole is necessarily prior to the part may be taken to mean that the predicate follows as an effect of a prior (efficient) cause. Thus, for example, in the event that a brick falls from a chimney we express the principle that the effect is preceded by a cause in saying that the falling brick is caused by gravity. Here the part (falling brick) is not said to be identical with the whole (gravity) but rather is caused by it. The distinction, then, between the two senses of the notion that the whole necessarily precedes the part is based on the distinction between essence and cause. For a further discussion of this distinction and its origin in the philosophy of Leibniz see Heidegger, *Metaphysical Foundations of Logic*, pp. 52-56, 109-117.

[54] See SW Vol. 1, p. 331.

[55] This account is generally referred to as Kant's deduction of the categories. Hegel uses this terminology, but he refers to something more than either or both of the deductions identified by Kant in his First and Second Editions. More important for Hegel is the so-called "transcendental schematism" in which the transcendental imagination provides a "schema" to combine the otherwise heterogenous categories and sensible manifold. The schemata of the imagination, however, are "nothing but *a priori* determinations of time in accordance with rules." Thus time

emerges as that "third something" which, being both intelligible and sensible, provides both the understanding and intuition their objective determination. See, CPR pp. 180-87.

[56]See SW Vol. 1, p. 332.

[57]See ibid. p. 332f.

[58]See ibid. p. 333f.

[59]We here skip over a long discussion (pp. 336-355) of the relation of the temporal and the eternal in the philosophy of Spinoza. The matter is of no little consequence to Hegel, but, since the text itself involves Hegel's criticism of Jacobi's criticism of Spinoza's thought, it can well be left aside as too intricate.

[60]See ibid. p. 363.

[61]See ibid. p. 373.

[62]See ibid. p. 378.

[63]See ibid. p. 379f.

[64]See ibid. p. 384f.

[65]See ibid. p. 385f.

[66]See ibid. p. 386.

[67]See ibid. p. 387.

[68]See ibid. p. 388.

[69]See ibid. p. 392f.

[70]Ibid. p. 395.

[71]See ibid. p. 406.

[72]Ibid. p. 407.

[73]Ibid. p. 396f.

[74]Perhaps the most accessible statement of the initial process of abstraction is the following: Think of yourself, frame the concept of yourself; and notice how you do it. See Fichte, The *Science of Knowledge*, p. 33.

[75]SW Vol. 1, p. 399.

[76]Ibid. pp. 397ff.

[77]Ibid. p. 405f.

[78]See ibid. p. 410.

[79]See ibid. p. 432f.

[80]Ibid. p. 433.

[81]See the introduction to *Religion within the Limits of Reason Alone*, trans. Theodore M. Greene and Hoyt H. Hudson (New York: Harper & Brothers, 1960) p. xxxivf.

[82]An adequate account of the affair can be found in the *Encyclopedia of Philosophy*, gen. ed. Paul Edwards, Vol. 1, (New York: Macmillan Publishing Co., Inc. & The Free Press, 1967) pp. 189-192 under the heading "Atheismusstreit".

[83]See the article on Jacobi in the *Encyclopedia of Philosophy*, Vol. 4, pp. 235-238.

6

THE ESSAY ON NATURAL LAW[1]

The publication of the *Critical Journal of Philosophy* broke off suddenly and unexpectedly in May of 1803 when Schelling left Jena. Plans were in the offing for continuing the journal despite Schelling's absence, but these never materialized.[2] The essay on natural law was thus Hegel's last contribution to the cause.

This turn of events warrants a pause. Hegel had spent the last two years furiously composing his attacks upon the philosophy of the day. True to his intentions he had begun to lay the philosophical heavyweights low with unrelenting criticism of the ideas and presuppositions of their respective systems. And, as we have seen, his campaign had not been a haphazard one. Much rather he had followed a carefully devised hermeneutical strategy of demonstrating a systematic connection between the high-flown critical philosophy of reflection and its more humble cousin, common sense philosophy. Hegel exposed empiricism to be the common ground of these widely divergent trends in thinking by introducing the element of scepticism. The thoroughgoing denial of experience which characterizes genuine scepticism for Hegel represented the common foe of both philosophical movements. Thus the philosophy of common sense fled from scepticism into the illusory sanctuary of experience, while the more sophisticated philosophy of reflection fled into an ideal beyond posited as the abstraction from experience. Accordingly, whether an appeal was made to mere empirical knowledge or to the lofty ideal of faith, still there was involved the basic flight from the nullity of scepticism.

In the article on faith and knowledge Hegel portrayed the incapacity to face the nothingness of understanding as leading to the feeling that God is dead. For, in attempting to maintain the objectivity of the understanding, the reflection-philosophy was led to renounce reason and its proper manifestation in thinking. The consequence was to deny the identity of thinking and being truly expressed in the proposition that God exists.

175

As the highest truth of philosophy[3] this idea represents the Absolute. Yet even as absolute this idea is manifest in the many parts which comprise the singular whole of philosophy. As such its truth can be discovered, not only within the bounds of philosophy proper, but also in all other genuine sciences. The science of natural law was one such manifestation of the Absolute, and so warranted the attention of the young Hegel.

When taken in its context of the *Critical Journal of Philosophy*, therefore, the essay on natural law is seen to be Hegel's first attempt to expropriate the idea of philosophy for grasping the sphere of human action in the world. That this subject was of special importance to Hegel goes without saying. Philosophy must be made to speak to human needs and desires, if it is not to be lifeless and cold. But it is equally the case that the science of natural law is, in Hegel's view, but one of the many shapes that the idea must necessarily take up. Accordingly, the sudden abandonment of the *Critical Journal of Philosophy* should be seen as an accident of human affairs that curtailed the full exposition of the idea of philosophy.

One could well imagine that, if Schelling had not left his colleague in the lurch, Hegel would have continued to compose essays expounding the positive consequences of his interpretation of philosophy in his native Germany.[4] Instead he seems to have been thrown into confusion and doubt about the purpose of his writings, and so he lay down his pen, only to resume his published compositions when he had established the outlines of his own philosophical system four years later in the *Phenomenology*.

The point here is not to make Schelling out as the scapegoat, blaming him for Hegel's failed ideal. It is rather to show that Hegel had built up a considerable head of steam in writing his contributions to the *Critical Journal of Philosophy* only to have it suddenly dissipate. Thus the essay on natural law will be taken as the first, if only actual, installment in a journal that was to be no longer predominantly critical in its approach, but rather a positive contribution to the unified idea of philosophy. The antecedent *Glauben und Wissen* is then seen to be the true watershed of this period, defining the difference between pure criticism and pure speculative thinking, and establishing the hermeneutical imperative of philosophy. The positive advance made on the science of natural law in the article here under consideration must therefore be read in light of the pronouncement of the death of God.

Hegel's comments on natural law stem neither from the philosophy of reflection nor from the pre-critical dogmatism of common sense. Much rather their origin lies in a post-critical consideration of the sphere of human action, in a perspective of thinking that post-dates the death of God. Hegel's guiding question in this essay may thus be formulated as follows: What is the truth of the world, now that God is dead?

This is not obvious to one who merely takes up with the essay on natural law, and begins to read it from the first word to the last. For the first part of the essay immediately resumes the discussion of common sense philosophy and critical reflection, even if under the guise of ethics. But even as ethics here emerges as the overriding concern of the young philosopher so too does the reality of history. And this is where the real difference in this essay lies. For here Hegel considers the fatefulness of history that was foreshadowed in the utterance that God is dead.

Ethics, for Hegel, is a human historical necessity. This necessity, however, does not stem from the arbitrary and accidental course of human events, but rather from the exigencies of the Absolute Idea upon human thinking. Thus the consideration of the common sense approach to ethics, on one hand, and the reflective treatment of ethics, on the other, is immersed in the issue of the fate of human historical thinking and existence. The criticism of these approaches to the subject of ethics is thus infused with a sense of the necessity of the Absolute Idea as it is played out in history. It is for this reason that the manifestly critical first part of the essay is followed with an original analysis of comedy and tragedy that illuminates the full coincidence of the philosophical Idea and the science of natural law, of thinking and being, and of life and death.

The essay on natural law begins with the supposition that the Idea must necessarily take shape, in part, in natural law. But, Hegel argues, the science of natural law has shared the fate of other sciences, such as mechanics and physics, in being divorced from what is philosophical in philosophy. Metaphysics has taken philosophy out of the hands of the sciences, and so it has divorced the sciences from the Idea. Experience has stepped into the void left by philosophy, becoming the new principle which guides the development of science. Accordingly, science has become a mere collection of empirical observations, strung together by various concepts or by the categories of the understanding.[5]

Despite this state of affairs, Hegel maintains, every science is capable of acquiring its own inner necessity. If a science be taken as a part of philosophy, as a part of the absolute whole, it becomes genuinely scientific. But even as various sciences are developed as parts of the whole, the Idea itself remains free from the determination of the given science. The particular sciences reflect the Idea, but do not exhaust it:

> But the Idea itself remains free of this determinacy and it can be reflected in this determinate science just as purely as absolute life is expressed in every living thing. (*Natural Law*, trans. T.M. Knox [University of Pennsylvania Press, 1975], p. 55)

Any given science is, in Hegel's analysis, only an image of the Idea, and so must be distinguished from the absolute science of philosophy, which makes use of the pure form of the Idea. The preeminent example of a science that reflects the image of the Idea is geometry. As such we see in geometry a self-standing and complete image of the Idea, expounded through intuition, independent of the constricting influence of concepts.[6]

In order for a given science to become a perfect reflection of the Idea, Hegel argues, intuition, image, and concept must be unified and taken up into the ideal.[7] But also, and more importantly, the science must be stripped of its separateness; its principle must be realized in its higher context and necessity (in the Idea), and thus be completely freed (from the limitations of the understanding).[8] Thus not only universal knowledge is required for genuine science, but also the freedom granted by the Idea.

The synthesis of intuition, image, and concept in science has been accomplished, according to Hegel, in the Critical philosophy (of Kant). But this advance, though crucial, is negative in character:

> The Critical philosophy has had the important *negative* effect on theoretical sciences of proving that the scientific element in them is not objective, but belongs to a middle realm between nothing and reality, to a mixture of being and not-being, and thus making them admit that they belong only to the sphere of empirical thinking. (Ibid. p. 57)

It is because of the mixture of common sense empiricism and scepticism involved here that Hegel maintains science is at most an image of the Idea, rather than the truth about the thing in-itself. The step is a crucial one, because it prepares for the liberation of science for the Idea by demonstrating that understanding as such grants only limited knowledge, or knowledge limited by the understanding to appearance.

However, the Critical philosophy has failed, in Hegel's judgment, to liberate science from the understanding, and so its positive effect has amounted to nothing. For, being incapable of overcoming the inherent opposition of concept and intuition in appearance, it has fallen short of their absolute identity in the Idea.[9]

Hegel argues that, because all previous treatments of natural law stem from a conception of science that has suffered the fate of being divorced from the Idea, all ethical theories, present and past, must be denied the status of genuine science. All alike have failed to make the positive move to absolute identity. Instead they have only come so far as to become entrenched in the element of opposition (of concept and intuition, of universal principle and particular) and negativity (of empty knowledge and precepts). They have even failed to attain to absolute negativity (the complete denial of understanding). Such attempts at natural law thus remain a mixture of the positive (empirical) and the negative (logical). Thus mixed, these attempts have neither the purely negative nor the purely positive in their grasps which is an absolute requirement for attaining the identity of the Idea.

Hegel's interest in previous attempts at natural law stems from a twofold concern with the history of science. His first concern is to discover how the empirical condition of the world is reflected in the ideal (universal) mirror of science. The second concern is to compare these attempts at science to the Absolute Idea, and to discern therein how, even while dominated by the moments of this Idea, they necessarily distort it. Hegel's interest here in the history of science is thus informed by his supposition that the reflection of the Idea by science is fated to become a distortion.[10]

As regards the ideal (universal) reflection of the Idea in science, Hegel proposes that, all things being interconnected, empirical existence and the condition of all sciences will express the condition of the world. The condition of natural law expresses this pre-eminently, because it bears on the ethical, the mover of all things human. The science of ethics thus exists only insofar as it is one with the empirical shape of the ethical, and expresses that shape universally.[11]

A. Scientific Empiricism.

That form of science which reflects the condition of the world in the mirror of universal principles is, according to Hegel, empirical science. Here is found an opposition in the form and content of ethical knowledge. On one hand we have principles of action and on the other particular instances of action. The opposition of the form and the content exists as a relative coincidence of concepts and intuitions, for here the principles are nothing but abstractions of particulars.[12]

That ethical science in which there exists a necessary distortion of the Idea Hegel calls the formal science of ethics. Here is found an absolute opposition of form and content: the pure unity of the form (concept) is wholly separated from the content (intuition), and posited independently.[13]

What is common to both types of sciences, Hegel maintains, is the empirical. In the case of empirical science, the Absolute is a simple derivative of the empirical. With formal science, on the other hand, the Absolute is posited as an ideal lying beyond the reach of science. Thus even in formal science only the empirical is left as the object of scientific knowledge.[14]

Hegel's interest in the empirical science of natural law proper has a negative aim. Rather than taking up with individual principles comprising this science, and considering them in their interrelation, he proceeds to establish one basic point: the principles of this science are nothing but particular determinacies and relational concepts in abstraction. And, so Hegel argues, it is just this fixation upon such determinacies which must be denied in the science of ethics.

The empiricist approach to ethics, Hegel notes, begins with the concept of a given relation, e.g., marriage, and proceeds to explain this relation by fixing upon a given determinacy (procreation, common property, etc.), and claiming it as the essence of marriage. The consequence of such an empirical procedure is that differing determinacies will inevitably be posited as the essence of marriage, and a neverending quarrel over the hierarchy of determinacies will ensue. This struggle, moreover, can never be finally resolved, because as singular determinacies the principles of the science lack internal necessity. One principle can be held forth as necessary as easily as another. Furthermore, in empirical science (as contrasted with formal science) the transformation of an individual determinacy into a principle of science occurs unconsciously, and so does not become an object of reflection.[15]

Because the process of raising determinacies to the level of principles remains unconscious in the empirical science of ethics, the need arises to present the image of the absolute unity of the many various principles that demand attention, and thereby to establish the simple necessity of the science. Thus in the empirical approach to ethics, the absolute Idea comes under the seemingly insurmountable opposition of the one and the many. The absolute Idea accordingly manifests itself in the misshapen form of this opposition.[16]

The need for establishing the absolute unity of the multifarious principles of empirical science can, in Hegel's judgment, never be fulfilled. Since the empirical approach is rooted in a multiplicity of principles, which are in fact nothing but individual determinacies smuggled in under the guise of universality, no unity of principles is possible. The unity posited as the ideal of empirical science annihilates the multiplicity of principles and determinacies, and so eradicates empiricism itself. But, because this unity remains only an ideal, a residual empiricism must still be recognized:

> In that ideal, empiricism, in which what thus passes vaguely for capricious and accidental is blurred, and the smallest indispensable mass of the multiplex is posited; it is *chaos* in the physical as in the ethical world. Chaos in the latter is conceived now by the imagination more in the image of existence, as the *state of nature*, now by empirical psychology more in the form of potentiality and abstraction, as a list of the capacities found in man, as the *nature and destiny of man*. (Ibid. p. 63)

However, it is, according to Hegel, contradictory to conceive of the ethically necessary as the state of nature or as the nature and destiny of humankind and then to posit this chaos as a fiction or as a mere possibility. Hegel notes further that even the postulate of a divine origin for ethical chaos grants no way out of the morass of empiricism, since this empiricism precludes the absolute unity of the one (God) and the many (chaos).[17] In the end the struggle to establish a consistent image of absolute unity amidst the chaos of the ethical world leads to the piecemeal rejection and nullification of certain experiences and determinacies in lieu of certain others. The consequence is that perception of the empirical is distorted. Rather than perceiving the organic totality of the world, a skewed perspective, based on established moral prejudices, is claimed for experience. Hegel proposes that, in order to counter this influence upon experience, it is necessary to reintroduce the true inconsistency of empiricism in which each thing counts for perception as much as the other. Hegel introduces this basic conception of experience by distinguishing pure empiricism from scientific empiricism.[18]

B. Pure Empiricism.

Pure empiricism is characterized by its thoroughgoing inconsistency, and is justified in this inconsistency by the nature of experience itself. As regards ethics, pure empiricism can grant an intuition of the ethical life that fully reflects the Idea. So long as the intuition of the ethical life is withheld from the contaminating influence of the understanding (as found in scientific empiricism), it will bear witness to an ordered world, and thus to a creator. Pure empiricism will struggle with the concepts by which it must express its situation; that intuition will take on distorted forms in its passage through consciousness; it will be confused and contradictory in the use of concepts. Yet the arrangement of the parts and the self-modifying determinations of pure empiricism will proclaim the invisible but inwardly rational spirit. And, if this appearance be taken as a product and result (of the passage through consciousness), it will completely correspond with the Idea.[19]

Supported by its intuition of the whole, however turbid, pure empiricism justifiably rejects the science of empiricism. For pure empiricism provides scientific empiricism with the organic, living whole of experience, and the latter proceeds to kill this life by dissecting it into certain various determinant principles, and positing them as absolute.[20] However, according to Hegel, between the unconscious intuition of the ethical life and its expression in concepts lies a middle term, namely, consciousness. By passing into consciousness, such intuition comes into fateful contact with the concept: multiplicity and finitude are necessarily absolutely engulfed in universality.[21]

C. Formal Science.

The infinity and universality into which pure empiricism inevitably sinks is represented by formal science. This science is distinguished, in Hegel's treatment, by the absolute concept, or infinity. In formal science the mixture of the complex and the simple, of the many and the one, characteristic of empirical science is transformed into the complete separation of the *a priori* from the empirical. Especially in the idealism of Kant and Fichte the simple, the one, has been raised to a level of total abstraction and become infinity.[22]

Hegel declines to develop the notion of infinity that figures in his analysis of formal science, but he does make a few comments about it in passing. The essence of infinity, he notes, is that it is the unmediated opposite of itself. As such it is the principle of movement and change, undergoing manifold metamorphoses as it contradicts itself in its opposite. Common to these metamorphoses is the transformation of infinity into its contradictory. This transformation is the essence of infinity, and is called the absolute opposition between pure identity and pure non-identity. Pure identity is the abstraction of form, and pure non-identity is the absolute opposition of form and content. Thus as the abstraction of form, infinity is (as its opposite) also the absolute opposition of form and content, or finitude. Being at once infinite (as abstraction of form) and finite (as the opposition of form and content) the infinite is absolutely finite, or absolute finitude. It is in this respect that it is the principle of movement and change.[23]

The transition of infinity into finitude, identity into non-identity, can be stopped, according to Hegel, only by proceeding empirically to fix a given finite metamorphosis, and then negating that metamorphosis by abstracting the infinite from it. Thus the infinite arises as the negation of multiplicity (finitude), and is then deemed positively to be pure unity. The pure unity so arrived at is called pure reason.[24]

Pure reason, Hegel notes, has a double relation to the finite. On one hand it is the abstraction of unity from multiplicity. As such it presupposes the existence of the finite, even as it stands opposed to it. This relation of pure reason to the finite is called pure theoretical reason. On the other hand, pure reason is the positive unity which negates multiplicity. The negation of the opposition of pure reason and the finite is called pure practical reason. In pure theoretical reason the opposition between reason and the finite is maintained, and so theoretical reason is ideal. The opposition between reason and the finite is negated by their prior unity in practical reason, however, and thus it is real.[25] But, because practical reason pairs reality (the finite) with multiplicity, the unity claimed by pure practical reason can only be that of a formal ideal. For, we might elaborate, if practical reason is real, it is multiple. If multiple, its unity cannot lie within itself, but must lie in its opposite, namely, the ideal. At the same time, if practical reason is thus ideal, the real lies outside of it. Therefore practical reason must be thought of as a causality in which the real unity is related to the real multiplicity. But in this case, causality stands between the ideal and the real as a difference, and so the unity of the real and the ideal is denied to practical reason.[26]

Because the formal ethical science of Kant and Fichte does not attain to the absolute identity of the ideal and the real, it does not, according to Hegel, belong to the sphere of morality. No theory can be truly ethical that does not conceive of the Absolute according to its Idea as the identity of unity and multiplicity.

The ethical Absolute, according to Hegel, is the identity of the finite and the infinite. As this identity the ethical Absolute is at once the unity of the infinite and of the finite. This identity can thus be thought in two ways:

> ...the appearance of the Absolute is determined (i) as the unity of indifference and of the relation, or the relative identity, in which the many is primary and the positive, and (ii) as the unity of indifference and of that relation in which the unity is primary and the positive. (Ibid. p. 73)

In the former sense, the Absolute has its appearance in physical nature, and in the latter in ethical nature. The identity of the ethical Absolute is thus the oneness and indifference of freedom and necessity. And, since unity is primary in ethical nature, it is free even in its relative identity, that is, in its necessity.[27] If, however, this unity is thought, not as the essence of ethical nature, but as the necessary relation of freedom to necessity (as in the theories of Kant and Fichte), the necessity posited overtakes this freedom, and the Absolute is thought merely as negatively absolute, or as infinity. Here the real, multiplicity, the finite, are known as sensuousness, inclination, and the base appetites; and the ideal is the unity of reason by which the ethical subject controls and reins in the sensuous.

Hegel holds that, even though this relation of reason to the sensuous is universally recognized as the heart of practical reason, still it belongs to the one-sided relative identity of the infinite and the finite: the infinite is merely the opposite of the finite; the ethical is the mere denial of what is base. As such it has its origin in what is base, and so cannot be said to belong to the ethical Absolute. Indeed the formal philosophy of practical reason has, in Hegel's judgment, chosen the unethical over the ethical.[28] In Kant's philosophy of practical reason, for example, duty is posited as the form of the ethical. But just because it is the form, it cannot possess any content. Thus it lacks the ethical. The one-sidedness of this theory is apparent in the imperative: choose so that the maxim of your action be supreme law. The choosing itself involves a content, but the elevation of the maxim abstracts from this content.[29]

But, Hegel counters, the task of ethics is precisely to ask after the content of the moral law. Yet, in Kant's theory, to ask such a question is as ridiculous as asking, What is truth?

> When the question: 'What is truth?' is put to logic, and answered by logic, it affords to Kant 'the ludicrous spectacle of one man milking a he-goat and another holding a sieve beneath.' The question: 'What is right and duty?' put to and answered by pure practical reason is in the same position. (Ibid. p. 76)

Kant, then, has passed judgment on the principle of duty and right posited by practical reason.[30]

Since no content can be given in the moral law of Kant, Hegel continues, practical reason is not only somewhat superfluous, but indeed false and the principle of the unethical. For Kant's theory does not remain consistent, but instead smuggles a content into the moral law by raising specific choices to the level of rational necessity. But, Hegel maintains, the choices are arbitrary, and so anything can be posited as moral law. This, however, is to let immorality reign in the ethical sphere.[31]

Because the unity of practical reason is thus given a covert positive content, it does not remain true to the absolute concept, or infinity. The conflict which arises between the infinite and the finite in the mixing of unity and multiplicity continues *ad infinitum*.[32] In the philosophy of Kant and Fichte, for example, the unity of the essence of right and duty, and that of thinking and willing is made absolute. They thereby conceive of the Absolute as unity, rather than as the oneness of unity and multiplicity. Thus the one and the many are posited as equal realities, and the reconciliation of the two is known only as an ideal possibility. Hegel concludes that this possibility must be weighed against another:

> That pure self-consciousness, pure unity, or the empty ethical law (the universal freedom of everyone) is opposed to real consciousness; i.e., to the subject, to the rational being, to individual freedom. (Ibid. p. 84)

Thus, Hegel points out, the task of ethics becomes, as in Fichte's theory, that of compelling the actions of every individual (real consciousness) through the force of the general will (pure self-consciousness). But, since the general will is only real in its subjects, it must itself first be compelled by an individual (supreme) will. The question then is, How can this supreme will correspond to the concept of the general will? Either it must be posited as a transcendent will which compels the general will, and in turn is itself compelled by the general will (a position which Hegel does not attribute to Fichte), or it must be posited as an immanent will that alternately compels and is compelled by the general will. This latter is, according to Hegel, the presupposition of Fichte's ethical theory. The power of compulsion is distributed equally between the individual and the general will, and no recourse to a transcendent will is necessary.[33]

Hegel counters that, if the power of compulsion is distributed equally between the individual and the general will, the result is equilibrium. All activity of the will is negated; there is neither action nor reaction.[34] In order to escape this ethical *perpetuum quietum* Fichte's theory draws a distinction: actual power belongs to the government, as the body of the general will; possible power, however, lies in the hands of the people, as the spirit of the general will. The actual power of the government is opposed by the possible power of the people, and the latter is thought to compel the former. That is, if an individual will asserts itself within the government so as to overtake the general will and to deny universal freedom, the general will of the people reacts by stripping that individual will of its power. This must transpire through a public declaration of the general will of the people, and not through the compulsion of the individual will by the general will embodied in the government, for this would be insurrection. The government as a body cannot constitute itself as a general will, because it exists solely as a mass of individual wills. Only by virtue of the spirit of the people can a community be established in which the general will is efficacious.[35]

This theory leads, in Hegel's judgment, to self-contradiction. For, he argues, in the event that an individual within the government seizes power and compels the populace according to his or her whim, the people have it put upon them to choose another individual who more adequately conforms to the general will. But, Hegel maintains, the populace is in no position to make such a choice. Uneducated as to the general will, the people are not driven by a vision of the whole, but instead by private desire. Thus the system is self-cancelling: the people are inclined to choose an individual will to lead them which is disinclined to act in accord with the general will.[36]

From these considerations Hegel draws the conclusion that compulsion is nothing in itself. Thus any theory of the ethical order based on relations alone (i.e., upon causality or freedom) is self-defeating.[37] The problem at the root of such theories, according to Hegel, is a mistaken conception of freedom:

> First, there appears the empty abstraction of the concept of the universal
> freedom of all, separate from the freedom of the individual; and next,
> on the other side, this very freedom of the individual, comparably
> isolated. (Ibid. p. 88f.)

Because of this supposition, morality and faith are sundered, for the moral sense
is crushed by faith in a supreme will that compels the individual will.

D. Absolute Ethical Life.

The proper definition of freedom, Hegel argues, begins with the proposition
that nothing is external to freedom:

> We must completely reject that view of freedom whereby freedom is
> supposedly a choice between opposed entities, so that if +A and -A are
> given, freedom consists in selecting *either* +A or -A and is absolutely
> bound to this *either-or* .... Freedom is rather the negation or the ideality
> of the opposites, as much of +A as of -A, the abstraction of the possibility
> that neither of them *is*. (Ibid.)

As regards the freedom of the individual, Hegel remarks that individuals differ
either from themselves or from something else, and so represent the indifference
of freedom.[38] He describes this notion in connection with the ethical Absolute.
The absolute ethical life comprises three moments. First, the individual is posited
as a specific determination, and is thus connected to the external, or the finite.
Second, the individual is abstracted from this determination, or the finite, and is
known as negative absoluteness, or the infinite. Third, the individual subdues
itself, forms a bond with its people, and thus takes on the shape of a universal
determination of the Absolute.[39]

The relation between the moments of the ethical life warrants further
consideration. The first relation is the abstraction of the individual from its
determination, the raising of the singular to the universal concept:

> But when his being is posited as individuality (i.e., as a negation
> positively insuperable for his being, as a specific determination whereby
> the external as such is held fast), then what remains to him is only purely
> *negative* absoluteness, or infinity ... (Ibid. p. 90f.)

This transition marks the advent of the negative absolute, pure freedom:

> But freedom itself (or infinity) is indeed the negative and yet the absolute,
> and the subject's individual being is absolute singularity taken up into
> the concept, is negatively absolute infinity, pure freedom. (Ibid. p. 91)

But pure freedom manifests itself in death:

> This negatively absolute, pure freedom, appears as death; and by his ability to die the subject proves himself free and entirely above all coercion. (Ibid.)

Death, Hegel says, is the absolute conquest (*Bezwingung*). And, because it is absolute, through death the individual becomes pure individuality. The individual as such and death are both cancelled in this conquest (presumably because the individual is no longer an individual after death, and death is no longer death without the individual). Thus, Hegel concludes, in death the individual is its own concept, it is universal.[40] That is to say, the being of the individual as individual is completely exhausted in death; the finite individual is its infinity; in death finitude and the infinite are cancelled.

The second relation of the moments of absolute ethical life is that wherein the individual becomes universal through membership in a people.[41] But that a people is one's own is manifest only in the risk of death:

> ... the individual proves his unity with the people unmistakably through the danger of death alone. (Ibid. p. 93)

And so, to risk death for one's people is to transform one's individuality into universality. At the same time, however, it is to transform the people itself into an individual: "...peoples, as individuals, take their position against individual peoples." Rather than being swallowed up in the communal being of the people, the individual belongs to the people in such a way that the people itself becomes an individual. This individuality of a people is manifest necessarily in both peace and war, when one people embraces or opposes another.

The relation of an individual people to another now emerges as the proper shape of the absolute ethical life. This relation has, according to Hegel, a twofold aspect. On one hand is the positive relation of peaceful co-existence. On the other is the negative relation of exclusion in which both peoples are posited as absolutely necessary:

> In war there is the free possibility that not only certain individual things but the whole of them, as life, will be annihilated and destroyed for the Absolute itself or for the people; and therefore war preserves the ethical health of peoples in their indifference to specific institutions, preserves it from habituation to such institutions and their hardening. Just as the blowing of the winds preserves the sea from the foulness which would

result from a continual calm, so also corruption would result for peoples under continual or indeed 'perpetual' peace. (Ibid.)[42]

The relation of the individual to an opposing individual, when the possibility of conquest by death is succumbed to, Hegel calls bravery. And bravery is the shape of the ethical Absolute. But this is not the simple bravery of one who runs a calculated risk for the benefit of others. Much rather it is the tragic heroism of one who risks not only his or her own death, but the total annihilation of life itself. Hegel fleshes out this possibility through an original analysis of tragedy.

Hegel analyzes the ethical reality of tragedy in terms of the reconciliation of organic and inorganic nature:

> This reconciliation lies precisely in the knowledge of necessity, and in the right which ethical life concedes to its organic nature, and to the subterranean powers by making over and sacrificing to them one part of itself. For the force of the sacrifice lies in facing and objectifying the involvement with the inorganic. This involvement is dissolved by being faced; the inorganic is separated and, recognized for what it is, is itself taken up into indifference while the living, by placing into the inorganic what it knows to be a part of itself and surrendering it to death, has all at once recognized the right of the inorganic and cleansed itself of it. (Ibid. p. 104)

The exemplary hero in Hegel's analysis of tragedy is Orestes, whose fate reflects the image of the ethical Absolute. Some explanation may be in order here.

In Aeschylus's *Eumenides* the story is told of Orestes' flight from the hounding pangs of conscience. The background of the drama is the ill-fated return of the victorious King Agamemnon from the Trojan War. Agamemnon is attended in his bath by his wife, Clytemnestra. Once he has cleansed himself from the gore of battle, he steps out of the silver bath, and into the waiting arms of his wife. She lovingly wraps him in a capacious robe of many folds. Then she strikes him over the head, and dumps him into his gleaming, watery grave. Orestes is the son of Agamemnon and Clytemnestra. After many years in exile, he returns home to Argos and slays his mother, thus avenging the murder of his father. The matricide acts under the aegis of Apollo, who apparently commanded him in an oracle to kill his mother in just retribution for the crime committed against his father.

The play opens in the temple of Apollo, where Orestes has lately sought sanctuary for the murder of his mother. But he finds no peace here, for he is dogged by the terrible Furies, whose ancient, chthonian office it is to pursue murderers to death. The conflict between Apollo, who sanctioned the matricide, and the Furies, who are driven in their pursuit of Orestes by the ghost of

Clytemnestra, is mediated by Athena. Orestes, heeding Apollo's counsel, flees to Athens while the Furies sleep. There he beseeches Athena to aid his cause. When the Furies arrive in a rush, Athena decrees that a perpetual court shall be established with twelve of her finest citizens to hear this and all cases involving homicide. The furies take exception at this infringement upon their ancient office, but, as they are in the house of Athena, the daughter of almighty Zeus, they concede. Orestes for his part agrees to abide by the verdict of the court, whether for life or death. The plaintiff Furies are the first to present their case, extracting a full confession from Orestes in the process. But this is tempered by Apollo's case, in which he declares that Orestes acted under the sanction of his oracular command. An argument then ensues between the parties as to the true nature of the crime. Apollo argues that the slaying of Clytemnestra is just retribution for her crime against her husband. The Furies maintain that, since Agamemnon and Clytemnestra were not kin, but Orestes and his mother are, the crimes are not equal: Clytemnestra's death has repaid her guilt, but now Orestes's death at the hands of the Furies themselves is required in recompense of his act. At which point Orestes asks rhetorically, Am I of my mother's blood? Apollo brashly answers the horror of the Furies by saying that a mother merely nurses the seed planted in her womb by the male, and so is not a genuine parent of the child. In proof of this point he invokes the case of Athena herself, who sprung forth full grown from Zeus's head. Athena, moved by Apollo's argument, volunteers that, in the event of a hung jury, she will cast the deciding vote in favor of Orestes's acquittal. As it happens, the vote is split, Athena places her white pebble in the urn, and Orestes is saved from certain death. The Furies are indignant, arguing that the verdict is a flagrant attack upon their chthonian office. Athena responds by granting them an immortal home beneath the perpetual court of the Areopagus, from whence they will always send forth fear as an incentive to justice. They are pleased with the arrangement, and henceforth become the Eumenides, bestowing joy on the just and heaping grief upon the unjust. The play ends with the proclamation that God and Fate are reconciled.

The *Eumenides* has a far-reaching significance for Hegel and his conception of natural law. The hero, Orestes, represents a crucial moment in the unfolding of the ethical absolute. His story, as laid down in the words of Aeschylus, is indeed the poetic depiction of truth and reality itself. Orestes kills his mother to avenge the death of his father. He says Apollo told him to do it. Nevertheless, the Furies hound him for spilling the blood of his kin. When he stands trial in Athens, the jury is hung, but Athena decides in favor of Apollo. Her judgment acquits the matricide, but also includes provisions that the Furies (the embodiment of the feminine and the hearth) should have a permanent place of divine veneration beneath the court. They will, it is relayed, be assuaged in their terrible grief by the sight of Athena on the Acropolis. Hegel maintains that this represents the cycle of objectification, destruction and preservation of the Absolute.:

> This is nothing else but the performance, on the ethical plane, of the tragedy which the Absolute eternally enacts with itself, by eternally giving birth to itself into objectivity, submitting in this objective form to suffering and death, and rising from its ashes into glory. (Ibid. p. 104)

But, we might have reservations as this point. Orestes is not destroyed, he is acquitted. Neither are the Furies destroyed, nor are Apollo, the Aereopagus or Athens itself. What, then, is the brush with 'death'? This much might be ventured. The Furies represent the domestic, the sphere of blood relations, in the Greek world. Orestes killed his mother, and so he infringed upon the sancticty of death and ancestor worship. It is for this reason that the Furies hound him. They would run him to death (we moderns must wonder whether this were a magical death). But he manages to escape while they are sleeping. He flees to Athens. Apollo defends him in the court against the death penalty (again, we moderns wonder whether this means an execution, blood for blood, or sorcery). Apollo's argument is based on the premise that Orestes' kinship tie to his mother is ineffectual. The seed was planted in Clytemnestra's womb by Agamemnon. The ultimate tie is through the father. And because Orestes was commanded, seemingly by the oracle of Apollo, to kill his mother, he did not commit a crime. It seems Apollo is making an argument that Orestes was the vehicle of capital punishment. Afterall, Agamemnon was a king, and so his murder is of a different order than that of Clytemnestra. Orestes, then, was the arm of the law. The twelve worthy citizens of Athens could not make up their minds about this. The jury cast a split ballot: six for the death penalty, six for acquittal. Athena, however, had already indicated that she would serve as the tie-breaker. She cast her vote in favor of acquittal. What happened here?

Hegel suggests that the contest between kin and god, Eumenides and Apollo, had been decided in favor of god. Thus Athens, as the embodiment and realization of the state (*polis*), had chosen in favor of the state. This act renders Athens divine and the muderous act of Orestes an act of divine justice. Orestes is thus delivered from the pangs of conscience and the certain death it entails. He is also delivered from the rule of blood revenge based on kinship ties. In the denouement of the tragedy, then, it is apparent that Orestes has risked his very life for the sanctity of the state. Let us reflect a moment on the quality of this life.

Hegel concludes that Orestes is delivered from the law of death-by-revenge, delivered from the very law of nature. In the same measure, he has been promoted (though I find it hard to say, resurrected) into the life of the state. This life is, to be sure, universal, as it represents in fact and in words the temporal appearance of the union of the divine Apollo and the mortal Eumenides. But this life no longer belongs to Orestes. It belongs now to Athena. Orestes lost his life as a private individual, as a member of a family, and gained the life of a citizen. It seems Hegel would have it that Orestes has overcome natural death, and now serves the master of immortal demise. But this is a tough thought. What does immortal death mean? I can only offer at this juncture that natural existence is replaced with civil existence. And yet, negation being what it is in Hegel, Orestes will still die a natural death. It is just that his death will now bear the mark of civil obedience. It will be a universal death. It will be, in a very real sense, the death of Athens itself. Surely he will merit a state funeral and a play or two to make his memory indelible in human speech.

Now the correllary. It would seem that anyone who risks his or her life by defying the claims of the family (domestic violence is most stringently ruled out!) is 'resurrected' into the universal life of the state. But let us note this is not the Christian notion of resurrection. This does not promise that one will rise from the grave to reclaim one's body in the hereafter. Hegel is clear about this at least. One still has a body, and that body is mortal and subject to all of the laws of nature and decay. It is the spirit of one that is 'resurrected', even if this occurs before natural death. The philosophical reason for this is that God has died, and no mortal will escape this fate.

But, considered in this respect, tragedy remains alien, a story about the struggle of a divine being for its life. Surely the mortal may attempt to imitate the divine, but this is not easy. According to Hegel, the divine nature remains something alien to the individual; the story that is enacted in Greek tragedy as in the Christian Gospel has remained the story of another. As a culture, as a world, we have been unable to truly imitate the divine. Thus the absolute truth can only be yearned for through religion.[44] As the object of a national cult, God is, according to Hegel, the *ideal* absolute shape of ethical life.[45] Death, however, is the *real* absolute consciousness of ethical life.[46]

Hegel points toward the reconciliation of God and death in positing the identity of the ideal and real aspects of ethical life. Unfortunately, he does not explicate any such reconciliation here. Presumably this is because such an identity is presupposed by his treatment of natural law. This would at least be in keeping with his conception of reason. In any case, the essay on natural law[47] builds upon the proclamation of the death of God made in *Glauben und Wissen*: What is the truth of the world, now that God is dead? The answer Hegel seems to intuit is that the world finds its truth in facing death as the freedom of the individual to be more than an individual, to be one with a people, to risk absolute annihilation. As it has been with God, so too must it be for all peoples. This is the consequence of placing the world under the aegis of "Speculative Good Friday."

ENDNOTES

[1]The phrase, natural law, may be somewhat misleading here. Hegel's concern is not with the laws of nature but with civil law. The phrase, natural law, is the traditional translation of the term, *Naturrecht*, which expresses Hegel's basic assumption that law is not *sui generis* but a second-order response to the needs of nature. The German title of the article is *Über die wissenschaftlichen Behandlungsarten des Naturrechts, seine Stelle in der praktischen Philosophie, und sein Verhältniss zu den positiven Rechtswissenschaften* (see SW Vol. 1, pp. 435-547).

[2]See GW Vol. IV, p. 536.

[3]Hegel does not simply propose a theistic philosophy here. For, as was mentioned in the preceding discussion of common sense, Hegel also identifies the solar system as the highest idea of philosophy. Such apparently Spinozist juxtapositions have contributed to the debate, now two centuries old, regarding Hegel's conception of God.

[4]Harris takes another view of the matter. He suggests that the journal was abandoned because Hegel had begun to rethink his system at this point, and that the perspective of the journal was no longer in keeping with his thought (see Night p. xviiiff.) However, even if Hegel abandoned the journal to devote attention to systematic philosophy, still he maintained the fundamental idea that the Absolute is manifest in the many and various forms of thought known to culture. Harris touches upon this in the introduction to his translation of *Glauben und Wissen*:

> "The technique which he here uses for the first time, of making a series of partial visions criticize and supplement one another, is still an immature but nonetheless recognizable form of the method that is so impressively deployed in the Phenomenology." (Faith, p. 3f.)

Harris adds that *Glauben und Wissen* and the *Phenomenology* are so similar that the former appears to be a sketch of the latter. I would remark only that the similarity is more properly between the *Phenomenology* and the journal as a whole.

[5]See SW Vol. 1, p. 437.

[6]See ibid. p. 438.

[7]Hegel's term is the *rein Ideelle*, by which is meant the conceptual unity of the understanding found in the categories.

[8]Ibid. p. 438f.

[9]See ibid. p. 440.

[10]See ibid. p. 440f.

[11]See ibid. p. 441.

[12]See ibid. p. 442.

[13]Ibid.

[14]See ibid. p. 442f.

[15]See ibid. p. 444.

[16]See ibid. p. 445.

[17]Ibid. p. 451.

[18]See ibid. p. 452f.

[19]See ibid. p. 453f.

[20]See ibid. p. 455f.

[21]Ibid. p. 457.

[22]See ibid. p. 457f.

[23]Ibid. p. 458.

[24]See ibid.

[25]See ibid. p. 458f.

[26]Ibid. p. 460.

[27]Ibid. p. 461.

[28]Ibid. p. 463.

[29]Ibid. p. 464.

[30]Hegel speaks of Kant "passing judgment" upon the truth of the ethical life. As is made clear when Hegel returns to this matter in his *Logik* (see SW Vol. 5, pp. 4, 27), the allusion is to the Biblical account of Jesus' appearance before Pilate. In the narrative Jesus claims that whoever is of the truth shall hear his voice. Pilate asks, What then is truth? and gives Jesus over to the people to receive his crucifixion (see John 18:38). It would seem that, to Hegel, Kant had done the same thing with truth.

[31]SW Vol. 1, p. 468.

[32]Ibid. p. 473.

[33]See ibid. p. 477f.

[34]See ibid. p. 478.

[35]See ibid. p. 479f.

[36]See ibid. p. 480.

[37]Ibid. p. 475f.

[38]Ibid. p. 483.

[39]See ibid. pp. 483-486.

[40]Ibid. p. 484.

[41]Ibid. p. 486.

[42]The allusion is to Kant's essay, *Zum ewigen Frieden: ein philosophischer Entwurf*, Königsberg, 1795.

[43]"... this body, as body, remains in difference and evanescence, and through the spirit, beholds the Divine as something alien." *Law*, p. 104f.

[44]SW Vol. 1, p. 505f.

[45]Ibid. p. 514.

[46]Ibid. p. 505f, 514.

[47]I will decline from presenting a resume of the remainder of the article (pp. 515-537), as the discussion of the positive sciences of law adds nothing to what has already been reviewed.

CONCLUSION: HERMENEUTICS AND THE DEATH OF GOD.

This investigation began by asking whether the death of God provides a way of grasping Hegel's philosophical system. The answer, arrived at after an arduous journey through Hegel's difficult early texts, is an enthusiastic, though extremely qualified, Yes: the utterance, God is dead, is the linguistic paradigm of Hegel's philosophical discourse, i.e., his system. The argument marshalled in support of this thesis is something like the following. Speculative Good Friday is the celebration of the self-sundering of reason in history. The *Critical Journal of Philosophy* depicts a time in which culture, led by the philosophy of the day, denied the possibility of thinking the being of God. It thus fled into a form of religion based on the feeling that "God Himself is dead." Hegel saw in this saying the ominous sign of an emergent system of philosophy, namely, the science of absolute knowing, or speculative discourse. As a reader of philosophy, he showed how this was the case: the hermeneutical imperative of philosophy is to interpret discourse as bespeaking the death of God. As an emerging systematic philosopher, Hegel began to reshape the language of discourse into a paradigm of the new philosophy. The utterance of the death of God serves as that paradigm. Moreover, it is possible to trace the path of this paradigm through its formal and material permutations in the corpus of Hegel's writings. But this is to go beyond the limits of the present investigation.

Let us review the concrete findings before we pass on to less definite suggestions about the whole of what Hegel accomplished. The three elements which inform Hegel's utterance of the death of God were presented in Part One. We saw that Hegel was concerned with the interconnections of language, life, and learning. From his earliest days at the Gymnasium at Stuttgart, to his first years as a professor at Jena, and beyond, Hegel stressed the importance of bringing learning to bear upon life by exploiting the living spirit of language. Our reflections on language were drawn from the *Logic*. We began there because only in that work does Hegel treat language thematically. Yet we found a connection between Hegel's

195

earliest writing and the mature philosopher's notion that logic must be transformed through rooting out the formalism of Aristotelian logic (precisely by founding logic upon the coincidence of form and content characteristic of the German vernacular). Hegel's early interest in the multivalent and contradictory aspects of ordinary language came to form the basis of his so-called speculative discourse. He made it known that he wished to "teach philosophy to speak German". And this wish, we discovered, was tied to the death of God. The *Phenomenology* served as our guide. We found that in the *Phenomenology* each stage in the development of consciousness is given a specific logical and linguistic formulation. This theme breaks off suddenly in the penultimate section of the work. It is in that section that Hegel deals with the death of God. Thus we concluded that the proposition, God is dead, is the final utterance of language before it becomes fully speculative. Hegel's notion of a speculative proposition (from the preface to the *Phenomenology*) substantiates this. The paradigmatic example of a speculative proposition is the statement that God Himself is dead.

In general, we found that the consequence of Hegel's consideration of language is the supplanting of the role of formal logic in philosophy. Hegel returns to language in order to bring thinking and speaking/writing closer to one another. The product of this is a speculative discourse.

Under the heading of life, we investigated the biographical context of this incipient discourse. We found that this new form of language occasioned a change in Hegel's life. We learned here that the necessity of the death of God is the same necessity by which we know that self-knowledge is won only through self-negation, or death. Hegel's utterance of the death of God in 1802 was thus the occasion of his philosophical maturity. The first utterance of the death of God, we concluded is a watershed in Hegel's career.

In Chapter Two we analized the findings of Hegel's principle boigraphers with respect to this theme. We presented the reasons why others had identified this period in Hegel's life as being of special importance. Yet we could not agree with the description of Hegel as a religious reformer turned philosopher. Nor did we accept the picture of Hegel as a life-long systematic philosopher. Our argument was that Hegel's concern was first and foremost to understand and articulate the relation between learning and life. This in no way precludes that Hegel was at some time a religious reformer or a systematic philosopher. Yet it does shift attention away from the two mistaken assumptions that Hegel was born with a system in mind and that he never gave up the ideal of a religious reformer. The emphasis thus fell upon Hegel's concern to lead an ideal life, a life in which one's learning took the shape of the ever-changing appearance of the Absolute.

Hegel's ideal life was his real commitment to the project of culture, or *Bildung*, which defined his age. Hegel and Goethe were the leading influences on what others took culture to be. Yet these two men had very different notions of what culture was. For his part, Hegel conceived of culture as having its end in the death of God. His utterance of this truth was his first contribution to the project of culture.

In Chapter Three we investigated the matter of culture under the heading of learning. We learned that Hegel's first published essay, *The Difference Between Fichte's and Schelling's System of Philosophy* provided the occasion for Hegel to return to the principal occupation of his studies as a youth. That occupation was to bring life and learning together through a special form of reading, i.e., criticism. Criticism came to define Hegel's Jena period, and it provided him with the occasion to establish a critical point of view from which he would announce his coming system of thought.

Some of the essays Hegel penned while in the Gymnasium were reviewed in this connection. We found that they present a continuity between Hegel's earliest years and his Jena period; when Hegel set out as a critic in Jena he was tapping a stream that ran deep within him. Thus his contributions to criticism should not be passed off as immature or otherwise uncharacteristic of his thinking. Second, we suggested that the themes of the essays flow together in such a way that they shed some light on the utterance of the death of God in the *Critical Journal of Philosophy*. For Hegel's concern with bringing classical and traditional religious language to life seems to be tied to his attempt to bring a speculative efficacy to the terminology of the critical philosophy which had led to the feeling that God Himself is dead.

Hegel's essay on Fichte and Schelling emphasizes the unique notion of the fate of philosophy. Hegel argued that thinking is a living thing, subject to the vicissitudes of history and human freedom. He held that the spirit of philosophy took up residence in various systems, none of which suited it. He pressed for philosophy to begin anew, with a speculative program. This was the need of philosophy.

With the notion of the "need of philosophy" Hegel establishes his genuine conception of philosophical criticism. The only way to truly criticize philosophy is to tell it what it lacks. And the lack of philosophy is also the lack which gives rise to the problem of culture. The opposition of subject and object in philosophy is none other than the division of learning and life in culture.

The need of philosophy can be fulfilled, according to Hegel, only through speculation. For speculation is that mode of thinking in which subject and object, learning and life, are united. And, if the spirit of philosophy were to dwell within the house of a speculative system, it would flourish. However, as Hegel notes, speculation and system are not co-extensive. Hence, the need of philosophy is finally a hermeneutical need. The spirit of philosophy must dwell within a given system, but it must also be liberated from its dwelling through critical reading. Hegel attempts in the *Critical Journal of Philosophy* to liberate philosophy from the grip of those systems which entrap it. This he does with a fully speculative and fully critical reading of the death of God.

In Part Two we summarized and commented upon Hegel's contributions to the journal. We established that Hegel wrote the introduction to the journal and four major articles. The introduction and the first two articles can be grouped together. Together they represent the stages of thought which precede Hegel's utterance of the death of God, namely, common sense and scepticism. In the article on faith and knowledge the death of God is dealt with as that which comprehends the identity and difference of common sense and scepticism. The last of Hegel's articles, on natural law, represents Hegel's first (and unfortunately only) philosophical installment in the journal that follows directly from the death of God. Thus *Glauben und Wissen* is the denouement of Hegel's critical contributions.

Hegel's concept of criticism is presented in the journal's introduction. The notion of criticism in Hegel's introduction is similar to that set forth in his *Differenzschrift*. Hegel established the purpose of the new journal as identifying and rendering clear the one and only idea of philosophy as it was represented in the scientific systems of the day. The sole significant difference between the two statements on criticism is that the one given in the journal employs much starker figures of speech. Here Hegel portrays the work of criticism as that of liberating spirit from the putrefaction of deceased culture. The conception of criticism employed in the journal is linked to the sceptical oracle that to philosophize is to learn to die.

Hegel's first journal article is *How Common Human Understanding Would Take Philosophy; Portrayed through the Works of Krug.* This article represents the simplest and most naive kind of knowledge to go under the name of philosophy, i.e., empiricism. Hegel criticizes Krug in this article for employing reason in a weakened sense in his philosophical system. Empiricism, Hegel notes, cannot do justice to reason. The empiricism here in question is correlative to the section in the *Phenomenology* on Sense-Certainty.

Next is Hegel's article on scepticism, *On the Relation of Scepticism to Philosophy; A Portrayal of its Various Modifications and a Comparison of the Most Recent Scepticism with Ancient Scepticism.* This article, representing the next level of philosophical development beyond empiricism, is correlative to the section of the *Phenomenology* on Perception. Here Hegel argues that modern scepticism has made itself an enemy of reason, and that it is the death of speculative thinking. At the same time, however, Hegel argues that scepticism is the negative aspect of speculative philosophy. Thus scepticism represents the self-sundering of reason. Scepticism's characteristic expression involves, in Hegel's judgment, invoking the ancient dictum that each word lies equally opposite every other word. Hence, scepticism employs contradiction in making its point. A conspicuous example of Hegel's, I remark, is that God has an essence which passes away in existence.

Then is Hegel's long article, *Faith and Knowledge; Or the Reflective Philosophy of Subjectivity in the Complete Range of its Forms as Kantian, Jacobian, and Fichtean Philosophy*. Here we meet with the highest form of philosophy Hegel criticized. Generally correlative with the section in the *Phenomenology* on Force and Understanding (as well as much else), this article criticizes Kant, Jacobi, and Fichte for presenting a philosophy that leaves us with the feeling that God is dead. Hegel's criticism is meant partly to blame these philosophers for this feeling, and partly to evoke it. For Hegel's article treats the independent and opposing philosophies of these thinkers as a single system which culminates in the feeling of the death of God. Thus, while Hegel seemingly puts these words in the mouth of another, he takes full responsibility for uttering what a critic must: the philosophy of the Enlightenment was such that the death of God cannot but come to speech. To philosophize is to learn to die, even if it must be God who dies.

Hegel's final article, *Natural Law; The Scientific Ways of Treating Natural Law, Its Place in Moral Philosophy, and Its Relation to the Positive Sciences of Law*, was to be his first attempt to philosophize after the death of God. He considers the philosophical issue of right from a perspective that has incorporated the death of God. The article can be read by asking What is the truth of the world, now that God is dead? The answer provided is that the world finds its truth in facing death, for this is the freedom of the individual to be more than the individual, to be one with what one is not.

Now let me offer a few observations about the gist of these findings. We begin with a strong note of caution. Nowhere did Hegel unequivocally claim the death of God as absolute truth. Yet we have seen how important this notion is to his understanding of philosophy and by extension culture. Thus the need of Hegel's philosophy is indeed hermeneutical: the elements of logic and life, thinking and being, from which his writing is constructed are most adequately conjoined through reading, and this under the aegis of Speculative Good Friday. The death of God must be read into philosophy. This is the truth of Hegel's system.

Let me suggest that it was through his articulation of the connections of consciousness and language, especially the German language, in his

Phenomenology that Hegel transformed the saying, God is dead, into the paradigm of speculative discourse. Here he led consciousness to the Golgotha of Absolute Spirit, that standpoint from which the systematic identity of thinking and being could be known. The speculative proposition is the form of this knowing.

In the *Logic*, then, we might propose that Hegel set his speculative discourse to work in axiomatic form. The speculative proposition can be seen as the paradigm of all propositions. Perhaps Heidegger's famous distinction between the apophantic proposition and the hermeneutical proposition in *Being and Time* has its source in just this paradigm. In any case, in the *Philosophy of Right* (and in his lecture cycles) Hegel seems to have exercised his speculative discourse thematically. This much is indicated by the parallel between the essay on Natural Law and the *Philosophy of Right*. But, one might want to cast the net even broader, and suggest that the death of God informs the material as well as the form of Hegel's philosophy. For the speculative proposition, God is dead, can enable us to think together the respective subjects of two great works, i.e., "God as he is in himself before the creation of the world" (*Logic*) and "freedom as death" (*Philosophy of Right*). The reconciliation of God and death is at once the presupposition and the conclusion of Hegel's system of discourse.

Therefore, we might venture the following with regard to Hegel's system and the death of God. The two major elements of Hegel's philosophical system are represented by the *Phenomenology* and the *Logic*. The *Phenomenology* depicts Hegel's narrative of consciousness, as it were, adumbrating the many and various stages thinking passes through in its engagement with the world. The culmination of this narrative is the total collapse of consciousness before the fact of the world, resulting in a way of thinking that is no longer based in consciousness as such. Self-consciousness, as the complete integration of what was formerly consciousness and what was formerly the world, emerges as that towards which phenomenology ultimately tends, but never attains. The *Logic* presents the surpassing of consciousness and world, the superlative alternative to phenomenology, the self-consciousness of God before the creation of the world. Thus the *Logic* represents that which the *Phenomenology* announces.

If, however, the *Logic* leads back to consciousness and the world, as would be indicated by the *Encyclopaedia* (Logic, Nature, Spirit), it nevertheless does not lead back to phenomenology. For, here what was formerly the subject of phenomenology is now the subject of logic; it is not narrative consciousness, but rather the necessary conjunction of thinking and being.

Finally, a brief word about how all of this is foreshadowed in the *Critical Journal of Philosophy*. First, Hegel's contributions to the journal fit together in such a way that we can with hindsight recognize them as a rehearsal for what later appears in the form of the *Phenomenology*. And, if the *Critical Journal of Philosophy* presents the subject of the *Phenomenology*, namely, the relation of consciousness and the world, in the form of the speculative criticism of philosophy, this only underscores the historical importance of that journal for understanding the later phenomenological work. For the course of consciousness limned in the *Phenomenology* is the more cogent when one realizes that its necessity is guaranteed, in Hegel's thinking, by the fact that the history of philosophy is the fated appearance of the Absolute. That the Absolute, the one and eternal idea of philosophy, submits itself to the freedom of thinking, that reason is the product of this submission, is nowhere more apparent than in the centerpiece of Hegel's journal, namely, the essay *Glauben und Wissen*.

The essay on faith and knowledge depicts a watershed in the history of philosophy, wherein the Absolute is seen to sunder itself in the opposition of thinking and being. This opposition is the breaking point of philosophy. It is that which is expressed in the feeling that "God Himself is dead," for here the incommensurability of thinking and being is felt as the impossibility to think God as the coincidence of thinking and being. Hegel utters this feeling as the "Speculative Good Friday". He thereby announces a speculative mode of thinking in which the death of God is seen as the fated appearance of the Absolute. Thus, in saying that the death of God must be grasped as a Speculative Good Friday, Hegel announces that the history of philosophy, and so too culture has reached a point of no return on the path toward the speculative union of thinking and being.

BIBLIOGRAPHY FOR THE DEATH OF GOD IN HEGEL AND RELATED THEMES.

Ahlers, Rolf. "Hegel's Theological Atheism." *Heythrop Journal* 25 (1984): 158-177.

Altizer, Thomas J.J. *The Gospel of Christian Atheism*. Philadelphia: Westminster Press, 1966.

_____. *History as Apocalypse*. Albany: SUNY Press, 1985.

_____. *Genesis and Apocalypse*. Louisville: Westminster/John Knox Press, 1990.

Birchall, B.C. "Hegel's Critique of Religion." *Man and World* 13 (1980): 1-18.

Brechtken, Josef. "*Die Wirklichkeit Gottes in der Philosophie Ludwig Feuerbachs.*" *Tijdschr Filosof* 35 (1973): 87-108.

Brito, E. "The Death of God According to Hegel; The Interpretation of Eberhard Jüngel." *Revue Theologique de Louvain* 3 (1986): 293-308.

Bruaire, Claude. "*Hegel et l'Atheism Contemporain.*" *Revue Internationale Philosophique* 24 (1970): 72-80.

Burbidge, John. "Man, God, and Death in Hegel's 'Phenomenology'." *Philosophy and Phenomenological Research* 42 (1981): 183-96.

Butler, Clark. "Hegel, Altizer, and Christian Atheism." *Encounter* 41 (1980): 103-28.

203

Cascardi, Anthony J. "Narration and Totality." *The Philosophical Forum* 31 (1990): 277-94.

Collins, James. "A Kantian Critique of the God-is-dead Theme." *Monist* 51 (1967): 536-558.

Cook, Daniel J. *Language in the Philosophy of Hegel.* The Hague: Mouton & Co., N.V., Publishers, 1973.

Corduan, Winfried. "Hegelian Themes in Contemporary Theology." *Journal of the Evangelical Theological Society* 22 (1979): 351-361.

Crites, Stephen. "The Golgotha of Absolute Spirit." *Method and Speculation in Hegel's 'Phenomenology.* Edited by Merold Westphal. New Jersey and Sussex: Humanities Press and Harvester Press, 1982: 47-55.

_____. *In the Twilight of Christendom*; *Hegel vs. Kierkegaard on Faith and History*, AAR Studies in Religion. General Editor Willard G. Oxtoby. Chambersburg, Pennsylvania: American Academy of Religion, 1972.

DeNys, M.J. "Mediation and Negativity in Hegel's Phenomenology of Christian Consciousness." *Journal of Religion* 66 (1986): 46-67.

Desmond, William. *Beyond Hegel and Dialectic: Speculation, Cult,and Comedy.* Albany: SUNY Press, 1992.

Dupre, Louis. "Themes in Contemporary Philosophy of Religion." *New Scholasticism* (Fall 1969): 577-601.

Duquoc, Christian. "Les Conditions d'une Pensee de Dieu Selon E. Jüngel." *Revue des Sciences Philosophiques et Theologiques* 65 (1981): 417-432.

Flay, J.C. "Religion and the Absolute Standpoint." *Thought* 56 (1981): 316-27.

Fujita, Masakatsu. *Philosophie und Religion beim jungen Hegel, Hegel-Studien Beiheft* 26. Bonn: Bouvier Verlag Herbert Grundmann, 1985.

Garaudy, Roger, *Dieu est Mort: Etude sur Hegel*, Bibliotheque de Philosophie Contemporaine. Editied by Felix Alcan. Paris: Presses Universitaires de France, 1962.

Gillon, L.B. "Le Dieu de l'Esperance." *Laval Theologique et Philosophique* 30 (1974): 55-61.

Harris, H.S. *Hegel's Development; Night Thoughts* (Jena 1801-1806). Oxford: Clarendon Press, 1983.

_____. *Hegel's Development; Toward the Sunlight* 1770-1801. Oxford: Clarendon Press, 1972.

Henrici, Peter. *"Der Tod Gottes beim Jungen Hegel."* *Gregorianum* 64 (1983): 39-560.

Hodgson, Peter C. "Hegel's Approach to Religion; The Dialectic of Speculation and Phenomenology". *Journal of Religion* 64 (1984): 158-72.

_____. "Hegel's Christology; Shifting Nuances in the Berlin Lectures." *Journal of the American Academy of Religion* 53 (1985): 23-80.

Houlgate, Stephen. *Hegel, Nietzsche and the Criticism of Metaphysics*. Cambridge University Press, 1986.

Inwood, M.J. "Hegel on Death." *International Journal of Moral and Social Studies* 1 (1986): 109-22.

Jaeschke, Walter. "Christianity and Secularity in Hegel's Concept of the State." *Journal of Religion* 61 (1981): 127-45.

_____. "Speculative and Anthropological Criticism of Religion; A Theological Orientation to Hegel and Feuerbach." *Journal of the American Academy of Religion* 48 (1980): 345-64.

Jüngel, Eberhard. *God as the Mystery of the World; On the Foundation of the Theology of the Crucified One in the Dispute between Theism and Atheism.* Translated by Darrell L. Guder. Grand Rapids: Eerdmans, 1983.

Kelly, Michael. "The Post-War Hegel Revival in France: A Bibliographical Essay." *Journal of European Studies* 13 (1983): 199-216.

Kim, Chin-Tai. "Transcendence and Immanence." *Journal of the American Academy of Religion* 55 (1987): 537-49.

Kojeve, Alexandre. "The Idea of Death in the Philosophy of Hegel." Translated by Joseph J. Carpino. Interpretation 3 (1973): 114-56.

_____.*Introduction a la lecture de Hegel: Lecons sur la Phenomenologie de l'esprit, professees de 1933 a 1939...* Edited by Raymond Queneau. Paris: 1947.

Krell, David. F. "The End of Metaphysics: Hegel and Nietzsche on Holiday." *Research in Phenomenology* 13 (1983): 175-82.

Labarriere, Pierre-Jean. "Le Dieu de Hegel." *Laval Theologique et Philosophique* 42 (1986):d 235-246.

Lakeland, Paul F. "Hegel's Atheism." *Heythrop Journal* 21 (1980): 245-59.

Lauer, Quentin. *Hegel's Concept of God*, SUNY Series in Hegelian Studies. General Editor Quentin Lauer. Albany: SUNY Press, 1982.

_____. *Hegel's Idea of Philosophy; With a New Translation of Hegel's 'Introduction to the History of Philosophy'*. New York: Fordam University Press, 1983.

Luther, O.K. and Hoover, J.L. "Hegel's Phenomenology of Religion." *Journal of Religion* 61 (1981): 229-41.

Masterson, Patrick. "Hegel's Philosophy of God." *Philosophical Studies of Ireland* 19 (1970): 126-48.

Min, Anselm K. "Hegel's Absolute: Transcendent or Immanent?" *Journal of Religion* 56 (1976): 61-87.

_____. "The Trinity and the Incarnation; Hegel and Classical Approaches." *Journal of Religion* 66 (1986): 173-93.

Nussbaum, Charles. "Logic and the Metaphysics of Hegel and Whitehead." *Process Studies* 15 (1986): 32-52.

Olson, Alan. *Hegel and the Spirit. New Jersey*: Princeton University Press, 1992.

Pambrun, James R. "Eberhard Jüngel's 'Gott als Geheimnis der Welt': An Interpretation." *Eglise et Theologie* 15 (1984): 321-46.

Pereboom, Dirk. "La Mort de Dieu dans la Philosophie Moderne." *Dialogue* 15 (1976): 92-112.

Perkins, Robert L. "Hegel and the Secularization of Religion." *International Journal of the Philosophy of Religion* 1 (1970): 130-146.

Rosenkranz, Karl. *Georg Wilhelm Friedrich Hegels Leben*. Darmstadt: Wissenschaftliche Buchgesellschaft, 1977.

Scharlemann, Robert P. "Hegel and Theology Today." *Dialog* 23 (1984): 257-62.

Solomon, Robert C. "Machine or Orgainism; The Root of Modern Atheism." *Frontier* 18 (1975): 163-66.

Surber, Jere Paul. "Hegel's Speculative Sentence." *Hegel-Studien*. 10 (1976); 211-30.

Sussman, Henry. "The Metaphor in Hegel's 'Phenomenology of Mind'." *Clio* 11 (1982): 361-86.

Taylor, Mark C. *Disfiguring: Art, Architecture, and Religion*. Chicago: University of Chicago Press, 1992.

Van Troan, Tran. "La Mort et le Probleme de Dieu dans la Pensee de Ludwig Feuerbach." *Revue Teologique de Louvain* 73 (1975): 304-61.

Verene, Donald Phillip. *Hegel's Recollection: A Study of Images in the "Phenomenology of Spirit"*, SUNY Series in Hegelian Studies. General Editor Quentin Lauer. Albany: SUNY Press, 1985.

INDEX